Dance/Movement Therapy and Sexual Abuse

Dance/Movement Therapy and Sexual Abuse addresses the vital role dance/movement therapy plays in helping survivors of sexual abuse.

Comprising ten chapters, the book describes assessment, diagnosis, and intervention techniques with child, adolescent, and adult survivors of sexual abuse. Using case studies, contributing experts in the field offer the reader a profound understanding of the therapeutic techniques related to movement and the body for the emotional treatment of situations of sexual abuse. The chapters delve into the healing components of treatment during childhood, adolescence, and adulthood, and combine psychodynamic understandings with body-mind theories, techniques from the area of somatic experience, and bio-energetic analysis.

Full of in-depth and comprehensive therapeutic interventions using dance/movement therapy to treat sexual trauma, this book will be an essential resource for dance/movement therapists and students of the creative arts therapies.

Einat Shuper Engelhard is head of the Dance/Movement Therapy M.A. training programme, a senior lecturer at the University of Haifa's School of Creative Arts Therapies, and lecturer at the Kibbutzim College of Education, Israel.

Dance/Movement Therapy and Sexual Abuse

Assessment and Intervention Based on Body-Mind Approaches

Edited by Einat Shuper Engelhard

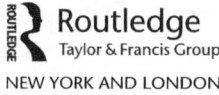

Routledge
Taylor & Francis Group

NEW YORK AND LONDON

Designed cover image: Getty Image

First published 2023
by Routledge
605 Third Avenue, New York, NY 10158

and by Routledge
4 Park Square, Milton Park, Abingdon, Oxon, OX14 4RN

Routledge is an imprint of the Taylor & Francis Group, an informa business

Library of Congress Cataloging-in-Publication Data
Names: Engelhard, Einat Shuper, editor.
Title: Dance movement therapy and sexual abuse : assessment and
intervention based on body-mind approaches / edited by Einat Shuper
Engelhard.
Description: First edition. | New York, NY : Routledge, an imprint of the
Taylor & Francis Group, 2023. | Includes bibliographical references and
index. |
Identifiers: LCCN 2022037124 (print) | LCCN 2022037125 (ebook) | ISBN
9781032312910 (hbk) | ISBN 9781032312903 (pbk) | ISBN 9781003309048
(ebk)
Subjects: LCSH: Sexual abuse victims--Rehabilitation. | Dance therapy.
Classification: LCC RC560.S44 D36 2023 (print) | LCC RC560.S44 (ebook) |
DDC 615.8/5155--dc23/eng/20221114
LC record available at https://lccn.loc.gov/2022037124
LC ebook record available at https://lccn.loc.gov/2022037125

ISBN: 978-1-032-31291-0 (hbk)
ISBN: 978-1-032-31290-3 (pbk)
ISBN: 978-1-003-30904-8 (ebk)

DOI: 10.4324/9781003309048

Typeset in Sabon
by KnowledgeWorks Global Ltd.

Contents

List of Contributors

Dor Haim, Maayan (M.A.), is a dance-movement therapist, DMT supervisor, certified supervisor, and bioenergetic analyst. She is a Graduate of Family Therapy certification program at Shinui Institute. Since last 28 years, she has been working at the Pediatric Psychosomatic Department, Safra Children's Hospital, Sheba Medical Center, Tel Hashomer, Israel. She has published several articles about eating disorders. Private practice in Tel Aviv, Israel.

Drori, Orna (M.A.), is a dance-movement therapist, DMT supervisor, and psychotherapist. She works at Merhavim Hospital-Medical Center, Beer Yaakov-Ness Ziona Mental Health Center. She works at Maor Center for children and adolescents who were sexually abused.

Etzion-Rosenberg, Orit (M.A.), is a dance-movement therapist, DMT supervisor and psychotherapist. She is running a private psychotherapy clinic specializing in sexual abuse, trauma, and inter-generational transference, as well as challenges related to sensual processing disorders (SPD), hyperactivity, and attention deficit disorders (ADD/ADHD). She also provides private therapy, group therapy, and staff mentorship in shelters for survivors of family violence, aid centres for victims of sexual assault, social services, and foster-care services, Psychological Educational Centres, Ministry of Defense, and the Multidisciplinary Center for Treatment of Sexual Assault and Incest Victims at the Bnai Zion hospital, Haifa.

Federman, Dita Judith (Ph.D.), is a dance-movement therapist, DMT supervisor, and psychotherapist. She is a lecturer and senior researcher at the University of Haifa's School of Creative Arts Therapies & Chulalongkorn University, Thailand. She has years of experience within psychiatric settings, children, adults and geriatric population. Her areas of interest are neurodegenerative disorders, trauma, chronic pain, 'mindfulness', and stress management. She has been developing her own form of 'attentive movement' with groups and individuals emphasising the relation between movement, creativity, awareness, and their relation to stress management.

Gottliieb-Eliaz, Einav (M.A.), is a dance-movement therapist and psychotherapist at Bnai Zion Medical Center, Haifa.

Gross, Orit (M.A.), is a dance-movement therapist, DMT supervisor and psychotherapist. Previously, she was a lecturer and supervisor in the Dance/Movement therapy Programme at the Kibbutzim College of Education and Levinsky College, Israel, and also Beer Yaakov Mental Health Center. Orit is a writer and creative artist, published articles in journals and lectured at conferences on topics related to the body and trauma, and published four books of prose (in Hebrew).

Maltz Schwartz, Ravit (M.A.), is a dance-movement therapist, DMT supervisor and psychotherapist at the Kibbutzim College of Education, Merhavim Hospital-Medical Center, Beer Yaakov-Ness Ziona Mental Health Center, Israel.

Nahor Michael, Sigal (M.A.), is a dance--movement therapist, DMT supervisor, and psychotherapist at the Ziv Medical Center, Safed.

Rosenblum, Ariela Lev, is an occupational therapist, B.O.T, M.Sc.O.T. at Ziv Medical Center, Safed.

Shalem-Zafari, Yifat (Ph.D.), is a dance-movement therapist, DMT supervisor, and candidate at the Israeli Institute for Jungian Psychology in honour of Erich Neumann. She is a lecturer at the School of Creative Arts Therapies, David Yellin College of Education, Jerusalem, and at the School for Society and Arts-Ono. She worked as the coordinator for the Creative Arts Therapies at the Jerusalem Center for Mental Health. There she established the unit for victims of sexual abuse and developed the dyadic treatment in the inpatient unit for mothers with postpartum and their infants. Counsellor at the Therapeutic Center for Youth at Risk-Denmark. Her articles have been published in journals around the world.

Shuper Engelhard, Einat (Ph.D.), is a dance-movement therapist, DMT supervisor and psychotherapist. She is a senior lecturer and head of the Dance/Movement Therapy M.A. training programme at the School of Creative Arts Therapies, Faculty of Social Welfare & Health Sciences, University of Haifa, Israel, researcher at the Emili Sagol CAT Research Center, and lecturer at the Kibbutzim College of Education, Israel. She worked as a therapist with Holocaust survivors and in various Israeli kindergartens and high schools with children suffering from emotional difficulties and developmental problems. Her articles, which deal with childhood trauma, adolescence, parenting, and couple relationships, have been published in leading journals in Israel and around the world.

Sichel, Yana (M.A.), is a dance-movement therapist. She works at child mental health clinic in (Ekhad Ha'am), Maale Hacarmel, Haifa.

Preface - Relearning the Body

Einat Shuper Engelhard

Introduction

About 20 years ago, I decided to volunteer at a centre for victims of sexual assault. I did not remain in the position for long. I felt alarmed. I remember my body cringing and being breathless when I was exposed to the abusive content. I felt that the sights and sounds were permeating my body and it was all too frightening and overwhelming. Even as the years pass, when I come closer to, delve deeper in, and try to know and understand those intolerable behaviours and abuses through therapy, research, and writing, the physical experiences I felt as I faced my initial encounter is the way of knowing, emotionally, occurrences that are unthinkable.

Sexual assault is tied to lack of judgement, to aggressiveness and to intrusiveness which create holes in the psychic envelope. Sexual assault breaches the body's boundaries, trust in another, normative processes of separation, independence, and enjoyment of the body. Sexual assault blurs the distinction between imagination and reality, impairs the ability of thinking, mentalising, and reflecting, it prevents daydreaming, playing pretend, muscle relaxation, deep breathing, pride in the body and its capabilities, its beauty, and in a safe relationship with another who sees, protects, approaches, and delights, and does not harm.

Healthy human sexuality is connected to love, respect, and equality and to a cloak of comfort and reciprocity. This book was written based on the body's life force, to try to become familiar with the ways Dance/Movement Therapy (DMT) aids in situations of sexual assault.

In DMT, movement is material for analysis. The patient uses movement as a means of therapeutic connection and as a way to communicate experiences which have not yet undergone representation. Observing the movement or joining it enables the patient to begin to think, jointly, about experiences that were, up to now, experienced in isolation and could not even be brought to the level of thought. In the treatment room, the patient chooses how and where she wishes to sit and which, from the moment of this choice, tells of the transference processes in the session. The therapist invites the patient to move between fragments of feeling and association interwoven in the body's motor abilities, and returns to the word which again invites movement and one more memory. The patient moves her or her body in any way they like. The assumption is that the associative-driven movement facilitates an encounter with particles of memory, feelings, emotions, and images, raw material that has not yet undergone mentalisation. The encounter with them in the body is the basis for symbolic thought.

The professional literature in the field of DMT for treatment of sexual abuse is still in its infancy. The case studies describe somatic counter-transference processes in therapy with children as a primary means of identifying sexual abuse (Ben-Asher, Koren, Tropea, & Fraenkel, 2002). Also described are the power of directing attention to appropriate and safe touch with sexual abuse survivors (Cristobal, 2018), and the contribution of DMT to identifying the boundaries of the body, reduction of tension, and attainment of a sense of freedom for children who were sexually abused (Ho, 2015). Other articles focus on work with women who were sexually abused and on the uniqueness of movement as a way to achieve a sense of security and connection to the body (Valentine, 2007). These assumptions were validated through qualitative research in which women who were abused in childhood participated (Mills & Daniluk, 2002) and who affirmed that DMT contributed to a rise in spontaneity, permission to play, struggle, freedom, intimate connection, and bodily reconnection. Other articles examine the uniqueness of DMT as a tool that can prevent sexual abuse in childhood and emphasise the advantages of movement as a method of learning about the body's boundaries, body awareness, and communication (Casey, 2018).

The different chapters in the book expose the reader to the various therapeutic approaches and diverse ways of work using DMT to treat sexual abuse. In all of the book chapters, the authors delve deeply into the healing components of the therapy. Unlike psychotherapy, in all the case descriptions presented in the book, the therapist does not only look at the body, feeling, thinking, and contemplating it, but also invites the patient 'to move her[1] self' and will often join in the movement. The genesis of an intermediate space for movement allows the patient to move what the body wants to experience and enables the therapist to think about the patient's need, about the movement emerging in the space and its symbolism. This is psychotherapy which encourages the patient to tell of herself through the body or to move everything that is in her heart, together with the words which merge with it. Body and mind, each supporting the disclosures of the other.

The book is divided into chapters according to the age of the patients and offers methods for movement diagnosis, assessment, and intervention in cases of sexual assault in childhood and adulthood. The first chapter discusses the uniqueness of the therapy in childhood via the theoretical framework proposed by Anne Alvarez (**Einat Shuper Engelhard**). The second chapter provides an answer to diagnosis and assessment questions which often arise in the treatment of children, in the face of non-verbal content which comes to the surface in the sessions (**Einat Shuper Engelhard & Yana Sichel**). The third chapter describes treatment in adolescence, a period during which sexual identity and gender perception are formed (**Orna Drori**). The fourth chapter deals with the uniqueness of the therapy in adolescence, in cases where eating disorders and sexual assault are both present (**Maayan Door Chime**). The fifth chapter describes a model for focused treatment of sexual trauma victims in a psychiatric ward (**Sigal Nahor Michael & Ariela Lev Rosenblum**). The sixth chapter delves deeply into the role of dance as a tool for processing sexual trauma (**Einav Gottliieb Eliaz**). The seventh chapter addresses assessment and intervention in cases of complex trauma (**Ravit Maltz Schwartz**). The eighth chapter discusses the in-depth treatment of a man and how intergenerational transmission of sexual abuse is revealed in therapy (**Orit Etzion Rosenberg**). The ninth chapter discusses identification of areas of change and emergence in the body's movement during the course of therapy (**Yifat Shalem Zafari**). The tenth chapter describes dilemmas which arise in processes of transference and counter-transference in the treatment of childhood sexual trauma, which impacts the experience of motherhood in adulthood (**Orit Gross**).

All the chapters combine dynamic understanding with body-soul knowledge, movement interventions, techniques from the fields of somatic experience, and bio-energetic analysis. The knowledge developed and constructed in all of the different chapters tells us that in the initial therapy sessions, movement intervention is threatening. The body, which experienced the assault, may reconstruct the attack or the experience of assault in transference processes. But, after trust and a sense of safety are established, the movement creates a space in which to contemplate and express embodied knowledge, and it presents the foundation for internalization of normative, healthy, preserving, and hopeful body experiences characteristic of safe relationships.

The chapters propose various movement intervention techniques, explanation of ways of therapeutic work, and an understanding of the significance of movement therapy in the context of the abuse. The authors' vast experience as clinicians is felt both in the singularity of their work and in the creativity and sensitivity and profundity of thinking and ability to be in an emotional experience, to identify it, and to verbally conceptualize it.

It is important to note that despite that fact that all the authors of the chapters work in Israel, by virtue of the multicultural nature of the population in Israel, the patients described in the book come from diverse backgrounds with respect to country of origin, nationality, religion, and culture. In the various chapters, any time cultural influences are involved in the cases described, explanations are given which detail the unique complexity with which they are associated.

The book offers explanations for dynamic processes that occur in the therapy room. It is vital to stress, though, that beyond emotional therapy, in cases where sexual abuse is suspected, first and foremost the authorities must be notified. We act to maintain the patient's safety outside the therapy room while the therapy provides a space for processing the trauma and for psychic growth.

Anonymity is maintained throughout the book in the case descriptions and pseudonyms are used. All identifying details have been totally altered so that the patients will not be exposed and their privacy will be strictly guarded.

DMT requires special training in which the body, movement, and dynamic understanding of bodily expressions are central. At the same time, I believe that the knowledge contained in the book will serve as an invitation to different types of therapists – to thinking and digging deeper into the knowledge in the field: arts therapists, psychologists, social workers, psychiatrists, verbal and physical psychotherapists, and counsellors and educators who wish to deepen their understanding of assault and its manifestations in the body.

Note

1 In the book, the language alternates between masculine and feminine, and the book's content is relevant to both genders.

References

Ben-Asher, S., Koren, B., Tropea, E. B., & Fraenkel, D. (2002). Case study of a five year-old Israeli girl in movement therapy. *American Journal of Dance Therapy*, 24(1), 27–43.

Casey, S. E. (2018). Moving to prevent child sexual abuse: Dance/movement therapy as primary prevention. *American Journal of Dance Therapy*, 40(2), 240–253.

Cristobal, K. A. (2018). Power of touch: Working with survivors of sexual abuse within dance/movement therapy. *American Journal of Dance Therapy*, 40(1), 68–86.

Ho, R. T. H. (2015). A place and space to survive: A dance/movement therapy program for childhood sexual abuse survivors. *The Arts in Psychotherapy*, 46, 9–16.

Mills, L. J., & Daniluk, J. C. (2002). Her body speaks: The experience of dance therapy for women survivors of child sexual abuse. *Journal of Counseling & Development*, 80(1), 77–85.

Valentine, G. E. (2007). Dance/movement therapy with women survivors of sexual abuse. In S. L. Brooke (Ed.). *The use of creative therapies with sexual abuse survivors* (pp. 181–195). Springfield, IL: Charles C Thomas Publisher.

Acknowledgements

I thank the therapists who took part in this important project – for their professionalism and generosity in anchoring therapeutic thinking, for their insights and the clinical knowledge they brought to the book and which are evident throughout. The chapters were written with sensitivity to the complexity of abuse and shed light on the special human connection created with the patients and on the intricacies of the therapeutic process which relates to the body and the soul.

Thank you to Judy Eichenholz for her professional assistance in translating and editing the main chapters of the book.

Thank you to my beloved family for their love and support all along the way.

Introduction
Coping with Trauma – A Body-Based Intervention Model

Dita Judith Federman

Introduction

This introductory chapter addresses situations of trauma and approaches to recovery. It presents the Movement-based Intervention Manual (MAMT) for Assessing and Treating Trauma survivors. The proposed intervention model is based on a study which explored bodily movements of trauma victims as they recounted traumatic memories, and on the practical implications of the bodily movement categories found to be manifest when a traumatic event is recalled. Evidence indicates a relationship between non-verbal expressions and the emotional, verbal narratives of a traumatic event.

R. sought therapy because of the anxiety attacks she was having in addition to difficulty sleeping; she also suffered from aches and pains all over her body. In the first meeting with the therapist, she told of the suicide terrorist attack she had witnessed and from which she was 'saved by miracle'. It happened on the high street of the city in which she lived. She suddenly heard a powerful explosion, after which she saw a bus erupt in flames. She later learned that 16 people were killed in the incident. At the time of the terrorist attack, R. was sitting with a friend at a café nearby.

She related that the din of the explosion caused her get up and for no particular reason make many spontaneous and useless movements. She wanted to run away but to her surprise, she saw something she had never seen before – her friend continued to sit as if frozen in place. Intuitively, she tried to hug her, to talk to her, and eventually almost picked her up from the chair and they left the scene of the carnage. Her friend was mute, did not issue a sound, while she, R., did not stop moving and talking. Images of the attack frequently returned to her in the form of flashbacks. She was looking for ways to 'retrieve that young woman, full of life' who had witnessed the incident. She wished to regain her body and soul and reach a relaxed place, a place where she could function, enjoy her body and enjoy the company of those around her.

This vignette exemplifies some of the somatic responses to a traumatic experience. Therapists see people who have been through traumatic events,

DOI: 10.4324/9781003309048-1

such as car accidents, wars, violence, and sexual assault. They are exposed to their suffering while providing them with source of support they can rely on, lending their bodies and emotions in an attempt to help in the complex journey of life in the shadow of the trauma. It is important for the therapist to address the question of how to help patients who have been through traumatic experiences to return to normal life. The therapist enables the body to 'speak' the trauma, and perhaps to even flourish, post-trauma. Thus, the difficult experiences can become supportive rather than inhibiting.

In ongoing crisis situations, the individual is, at times, not aware of the breathing, movement, or immobility taking place in her or his body. When the body enters a state of stress, survival response patterns such as fight, flight, freeze and even faint are observed (Federman, Zana-Sterenfeld, & Lev-Wiesel, 2019). In such situations, the person is 'stuck' or locked in a pattern from which it is difficult to disengage and yet, with which it is difficult to live a full and meaningful life. Experiencing a meaningful life becomes possible when a coherent emotional and conscious change takes place and the individual is able to shift from a survival-mode emotional state to a state in which he or she can experience the full range of meaningful emotions in the 'here and now'. A situation in which listening is possible – inward listening to the body and outward listening to the socio-environmental space.

Emotional dissociation is a frequent reaction to traumatic situations. Dissociation may be useful for coping during the traumatic occurrence but in the long run, manifests itself in difficulty identifying and communicating emotional experiences, feeling and describing body parts, or describing bodily sensations. Traumatic experiences impact the body activating the stress hormones and the amygdala, which in turn activate the fight-flight mechanism (the mechanism of the four F's: fight, flight, freeze, faint). Thus, the movements which occurred during the traumatic event continue to be reproduced/reconstructed and make the traumatic experiences feel as if they are occurring in the present (Van Der Kolk, 2021). In addition, the areas of the brain linked to speech and its comprehension, Broca's area and Wernicke's area, become inactive or unavailable, during the traumatic event (Van Der Kolk, 2021). This may explain the difficulty in expressing a traumatic experience in words.

Trauma is the body-mind system's reaction to a situation where there is an actual or presumed threat to life. It is a threat to the physical, mental, and social well-being of the individual or his associates. This can be a response to an acute event like death, rape, a car accident, or a sequence of events like wars, Holocaust, injury, and ongoing abuse (American Psychiatric Association [APA], 2013).

The consequences of trauma are complex and have far-reaching effects. They include varied and severe physical symptoms, physical illnesses, or emotional injuries that disrupt life. Phenomena such as flashbacks and terrifying memories will cause excessive arousal, constant alertness, and feelings of helplessness. All of these can cause anxiety, depression, isolation, dissociative disorder, addiction, eating disorders, as well as loss of identity due to the unconscious need to be separate from the body, the body that was the scene of the struggle (Afana, Pedersen, Ronsbo, & Kirmayer, 2010).

Approaches to recovery from trauma include: Medications aimed at suppressing overreaction of physical arousal systems, talk therapies, such as psychotherapy, which includes rebuilding trust-based relationships, and body-oriented therapies which invite the body to the possibility of emotional discharge and expression of feelings of helplessness, anger, and anxiety associated with the trauma. Dance/Movement Therapy (DMT), a body-oriented therapy, uses the body and movement in a quest to discover physical resources, and relates to the body's latent potential as a driver of the healing process.

Bodily movement is necessary for the process of recovery from trauma (Stromsted & Seif, 2015). The therapist's presence, adapted to the patient's needs, and taking into account the patient's movements during the traumatic event, along with the embodiment reflected in the encounter between speech and movement in the interpersonal [therapist-patient] therapeutic space, have the potential to change the dissociative space, and create movement within stasis.

Emotional regulation refers to the emotions that are felt, when they are felt, and how they are experienced and expressed (Gross, 1998, 2002). DMT summons/enables/invites emotional-physical expression. Patients are invited to express with intention and without judgement, emotions, and feelings in a protected therapeutic space. They practice breathing to reduce stress and find inner resources. They practice empowering body postures and movements such as wide, large, strong, and varied directions of movements.

In the trauma resulting from sexual abuse, the individual experiences a rupture in the attachment relationship. Such a breach impairs his or her sense of judgement and trust in others which may result in the formation of interpersonal connections that are out of control, and which at times include a connection with the abuser or with people who have the potential to inflict harm. The trauma of sexual harassment impairs the normal development of embodiment and the possibility of experiencing security and enjoyment in the body. This experience leads to helplessness, hopelessness, and even shame. The sense of stability and the ability to comfort oneself and for self-calm are also damaged. The individual will have difficulty 'standing with two feet on the ground' or receiving support. Since traumatic experiences are etched into the body, the body and movement become part of the solution, part of the healing process. With the help of the body, we can come to understand the trauma and know how to treat it. The fact that the body 'remembers' and can therefore be part of the solution is supported by theorists such as Van der Kolk, Peter Levine, as well as Pat

Ogden (Van Der Kolk, 2021; Levine, 2010; Ogden & Minton, 2000) DMT brings together body, movement, and creativity as sources for healing. The movement allows for a release of tension, an experience of sharing on a physical or pre-verbal level, and a sense of empowerment.

In a study of trauma victims (Federman et al., 2019), body movements that accompanied verbal narrative which shared either traumatic narratives or narratives of neutral events were evaluated. Results revealed three main bodily movement categories that accompanied the verbal narration of a traumatic event: **Illustrative movements** accompany speech and augment what is being said verbally. They illustrate *actions* and *emotions* and often, stand in for a word when it becomes too difficult to speak. For example: 'He held me so tight ……' or 'I was so scared, I could not breathe or shout'. **Rhythmic movements** are helpful when memory prevents expression of the emotion connected with the event. They express the person's natural flow of movement and are considered physical gestures, for example, moving forward and back in a chair when speaking of a traumatic event: 'I did not know what to do at that moment'. **Regulative and comforting movements** allow a sense of renewed ownership over the body, through repetition, self-touch, and cessation of movement where there was previously flow of movement.

The outcome of the study led to the development of a Movement Assessment and Intervention Manual, which uses verbal expression and movement and includes attentive movement, verbalisation, and embodiment. The model is presented later in this chapter.

The diagnostic method proposed here uses physical states manifest during and after the traumatic event (Zana-Sterenfeld, Federman, & Lev-Wiesel, 2019). The aim of DMT with trauma victims is to restore emotional and physical liveliness, rhythm, and flexibility. Since a significant portion of the communication is non-verbal, treatment focuses on non-verbal symptoms that accompany the traumatic experience and can be key in the healing process. Therapists often witness difficulty in finding words and in finding a narrative that describes the experience. Trauma victims report a sense of vagueness, they 'don't feel anything' they say that 'everything is alright. But looking deeper reveals situations of constant alertness, over-arousal, disconnection, or avoidance reactions.

In therapy, the encounter with the trauma of sexual abuse is particularly painful, even for experienced therapists. Therapists try to sensitively touch the deep scars that trauma leaves on the mind/soul. The DMT process encourages body awareness, thus enabling psychosomatic integration, aiding in the search for previously unavailable internal resources, and external forces that can be of assistance. With rhythm, creativity, tenderness, and interaction, movements that were available during the traumatic event are incorporated in the therapy. With the help of attentive, mindful movement, the traumatic stories are explored and processed and given a new, less threatening meaning, which allows for a different ending to the traumatic experience.

It is important to emphasise that the intervention model for working with trauma is a platform for therapeutic reference and not precise instructions for use, since in treatment the patient's condition in the 'here and now', their personal story and the special relationship between the therapist and the patient or group members are addressed. The model is suitable for trauma victims, as well as for those suffering from stress and anxiety.

The model for working with trauma describes four principles in the therapeutic process. When the treatment is group therapy, the meeting begins in a circle. Music and rhythm accompany the start of the session. This stage is defined as 'warm-up' to prepare body and emotion for the therapeutic process so as to create a relaxed, warm, and supportive atmosphere. Different parts of the body are activated to reach awareness of bodily sensations, of the space around us, and of our relationships with others, conscious movement is directed to patterns of flow, use of weight, time, and space (Laban, 1960).

The second principle offers an invitation to relaxation. Creating a place to relax, return to for rest and comfort when the pain is great. Techniques used are rhythm, breathing, and attentive movement which combines the principles of DMT and the 'mindfulness' approach (Kabat-Zinn, 2013). The use of rhythm is common to all cultures. Rhythm is transmitted in infancy from the mother to the child through the heartbeat and breathing, through a lullaby while being rocked, and a steady and soothing beat. These provide an anchor, a safe place to return to. The therapist, like the mother, helps in the transition from a chaotic-traumatic state to a state of relaxation with the help of rhythm. The rhythmic movement helps attain a feeling of being grounded and thus connects the body and mind to the present 'here and now'.

The third principle combines the search for internal and external (interpersonal) resources, physical and emotional resources. These resources can be obtained with the help of strong movements, grounding movements, exploring diverse movement options such as rhythmic dance in a circle that allows for a sense of control, self-confidence, and empowerment. Each individual has their own unique internal resources. A resource can be a physical experience that connects to the 'here and now' and can include internal sources of power, ability and control. An anchor can also be a memory of an experience accompanied by a sense of victory, success, power, and joy.

The fourth principle is the integration of physical experiences, feelings, sensations, and internal resources. At this point, the movements that were available or activated at the time of the traumatic event will be used again – illustrative, rhythmic, and regulatory movements (Federman et al., 2019), as mentioned above.

Comforting/regulating movements are soothing movements that allow a sense of renewed ownership over the body. These movements will be beneficial when feelings of anxiety and distress increase. They are usually repetitive movements or movements of self-touch/caress. In extreme situations when there is a feeling that it is impossible to continue, it is recommended that movement stop in order to rest. Therapist and patient will look for illustrative movements when emotional, verbal expression becomes difficult. They will practice a conscious exaggeration of comforting movements when the level of stress and anxiety is high. In situations of stagnation, the therapist and patient will together practice flow of movement.

The intervention model helps to release physical and emotional tension and allows for a reduction in the split between body and mind, thus allowing trauma victims to reconnect with their inner strengths. The challenge is to re-establish the possibility of experiencing security and enjoyment in the body, to restore to the body its vitality, rhythm, and physical and emotional flexibility. The advantage of DMT is the ability to infuse life into a body that is contracted, frozen, and/or immobile.

References

Afana, A. H., Pedersen, D., Ronsbo, H., & Kirmayer, L. J. (2010). Endurance is to be shown at the first blow: Social representations and reactions to traumatic experiences in the Gaza strip. *Traumatology, 16*, 73–84.

American Psychiatric Association (APA). (2013). *Diagnostic and statistical manual of mental disorders*(5th ed.). Arlington, VA: American Psychiatric Publishing.

Federman, D. J., Zana-Sterenfeld, G., & Lev-Wiesel, R. (2019). Body movement manual for the assessment and treatment of trauma survivors. *American Journal of Dance Therapy, 41*, 75–86.

Gross, J. J. (1998). The emerging field of emotion regulation: An integrative review. *Review of General Psychology, 23*, 271–299.

Gross, J. J. (2002). Emotion regulation: Affective, cognitive and social consequences. *Psychology, 39*(3), 281–291.

Kabat-Zinn, J. (2013). *Full catastrophe living: Using the wisdom of your body and mind to face stress, pain and illness.* London: Piatkus, Kindle Edition.

Laban, R. (1960). *The mastery of movement* (2nd ed.). London: Mac Donald and Evans.

Levine, P. A. (2010). From paralysis to transformation: Basic building blocks. In P. A. Levine (Ed.), *In an unspoken voice: How the body releases trauma and restores goodness* (pp. 73–96). Berkeley, CA: North Atlantic Books.

Ogden, P., & Minton, K. (2000). Sensorimotor psychotherapy: One method for processing traumatic memory. *Traumatology, 6*(3), 149–173.

Stromsted, T., & Seif, D. (2015). Dances of psyche and soma: Re-inhabiting the body in the wake of emotional trauma. In D. F. Seif (Ed.), *Understanding and healing emotional trauma: Conversations with pioneering clinicians and researchers* (pp. 46–63). London: Routledge.

Van Der Kolk, B. A. (2021) *The body keeps the score: Brain, mind, and body in the healing of trauma.* Translated to Hebrew by Iris Rilov. Israel: Pardes Publishing.

Zana-Sterenfeld, G., Federman, D., & Lev-Wiesel, R. (2019). The traumatic story as expressed through body narration. *Journal of Loss and Trauma, 24*(5–6), 400–417.

Dance/Movement Therapy with Children

Part 1

Dance/Movement
Therapy with Children

Chapter 1

Memory and Forgetfulness in Dance/Movement Therapy with Children Who Have Undergone Sexual Trauma

Einat Shuper Engelhard

Introduction

Children who have experienced sexual trauma carry body memories not recorded in the mind. In such circumstances, the trauma is expressed in actions, with no ability to speak it and give it meaning or interpretation. This chapter describes manifestations of the dissociation mechanism in childhood and the significance of attention and sensitive orientation to embodied knowledge, for achieving a life not governed by the trauma. The ideas of Anne Alvarez accompany the theoretical thinking throughout the chapter.

This chapter has been stirring within me for a good many years, during sessions in the clinic, in therapy, and in supervision. Encounters with a body that is restless even years after the trauma. All through the writing of this chapter, the work of Doris Salcedo (2007) has accompanied me. Salcedo is the Columbian sculptress who created 'Shibboleth', a 167-metre long crack in a cement floor exhibited in the Turbine Hall of the Tate Modern in London. The crack begins as a thin, hairline fissure, but as it continues, it expands and deepens, reaching about 60 centimetres. The work represents fracture in society, culture, or in the family. While reading about this work, a sentence spoken by Sir Nicholas Serota, director of the Tate at the time, made a profound impression. He pointed out that when the exhibition of Salcedo's work ends, the crack will be filled in, but its vestige, a scar on the floor, will remain and forever be a remembrance of it. The same is true of treating sexual assault, which is etched into the body and the psyche.

Dissociation in childhood sexual trauma

Sexual abuse in childhood undermines any grasp the child has of the perception of reality and normalcy concerning the boundaries of the body, privacy, protection, love, caring, tenderness, and pleasure. The body is unilaterally invaded and penetrated. In such situations, a dissociative mechanism is a refuge for the psyche, protecting it from disintegration

DOI: 10.4324/9781003309048-3

and madness. In the language of Bromberg (1998), the dissociation affords an escape in situations from which there is no escape (p. 242). This is the psychic parallel of the flight response when physical flight is impossible. At the physiological level, the hippocampus, responsible for thought, weakens and the amygdala, involved in 'sensory memory', works overtime.

When a child copes with an event in which there is an excess of catastrophe, with no one who can protect him, he disconnects from the experience with the aim of protecting his psyche's sense of continuity. The mind separates or splits off a part, as if it never existed. That part is not repressed – it is never even mentalised, represented, or processed (Gurevich, 2010). By not knowing of the event, partial control is gained over an extreme situation.

The intolerability of the event is tied to coping with contradictory emotions and conceptions (for example, a loving and sexually abusive grandfather). This is an experience which the child cannot think through mentally and still remain whole (Yarom, 2013). Gaitini (2020) compares this to poison kept in an isolated location, thus allowing the personality to continue to develop. That is to say, dissociation constitutes a defence mechanism and as such, preserves already developed parts of the ego (such as regulation, social competences, etc.) and safeguards the energy needed for further cognitive, emotional, and interpersonal developmental tasks in which the child continually engages. Thus, on the one hand, dissociation protects against complete cessation of development and on the other, this very protection is a barrier to encountering the trauma and processing it. And, without processing the trauma, the memories of the body, which experienced the event, still impact the child's functioning and are expressed through actions they cannot control, and in psychosomatic behaviours and phenomena.

This is not repressed material which, through a slow free-associative process, can be accessed. Many times, traumatic dissociative elements have not been mentalised, represented, or processed at all at the verbal symbolic level. Accordingly, the therapist's focus must diverge from language, which has rules and order; it must differ from the processing of an experiential narrative and should let go of the active search for content, memories, associations, transference, and counter-transference experiences, anything that is reminiscent of form (Gaitini, 2020). In situations where entering language spaces is not at all possible, the therapist must position herself, clinically, in a manner which commits to a regressive process in the mind (ibid.).

Therapy vignette

In just a few months, Justin will be graduating from kindergarten; this is his first time in therapy. He enters the room hesitantly, though from the moment his eyes detect the gouache paints, he approaches them with determination. On the paper spread along the wall, he paints huge genitalia; his whole body is excited, his muscles are tightly contracted, and his movements are quick. He giggles. The therapist hesitantly asks him to explain the painting. Justin throws the paintbrush to the floor and is swallowed up under a blanket at the end of the room.

Similar to the description of Justin, an encounter with perverted sexual content in therapy with children leaves the therapist unmoored. In such circumstances, therapists may confront the child with reality, ask about and examine the root of the behaviour with the aim of exposing the sinister secret in the hope of restoring sanity and saving the child from harm. However, not infrequently, the child does not know how to tell the story, to link, connect to, and restore logic and order to those unthinkable experiences.

In therapy, at times a suspicion of sexual abuse arises. In such cases, the responsibility for safeguarding and supervising the child's protection, outside therapy, should be placed in the hands of an additional external professional (another therapist or social-welfare worker). This will, along with therapy, enable an intermediate space in which the path to revealing and processing the experience is slow, ongoing, and critical to the continuation of proper development.

Due to the patients' young age, recovering from the trauma is complex. Not only does the trauma itself prevent reflective thought but at times, reflective abilities never had the chance to develop. Alvarez (1992) notes that frequently, due to the young child's dependence on and need of the abuser:

1 It is likely that the abuse or the abuser enthral him
2 It is likely that he is more afraid of the abuser than the abuse
3 Or, even the opposite-
   That the love for the abuser is stronger than the fear of the abuse

To perform the initial diagnosis regarding the manner of therapy, it is important to examine whether the child managed to experience healthy relationships prior to the trauma and whether treatment is provided close in time to the event. In cases where the answer to these questions is affirmative, it is likely that the damage will be at the neurotic level. According to Hartmann (1984), in such cases, the child can mentalise the content before it becomes concealed – a situation in which the traumatic knowledge turns into a block that cannot be pulled apart.

Under such circumstances, therapeutic work can and must focus on the memory of the trauma – in processing the experience, transforming terrifying and overwhelming material into content the patient can ponder and attach meaning to by providing a space to be angry, disgusted, hurt, and to share all this with the therapist.

In another situation, Alvarez describes chronic trauma in which the trauma colours the entire personality. Such situations take place when:

1   Trauma occurred at a very young age
2   Treatment was not provided close to the time of trauma
3   The child is not familiar with a healthy, non-abusive situation

In her article, *Child Sexual Abuse: The Need to Remember and the Need to Forget*, Alvarez (1992) notes that in situations of chronic trauma, the child can, in a slow process, begin to forget the trauma a little and build an aspect of his personality which is free of abuse. In this chapter, I suggest that therapeutic work through movement is related to the conditions which Alvarez presents as necessary for 'forgetting', as part of treatment of chronic sexual trauma in childhood. The first condition she presents is the need for space which facilitates 'remembering in parts'.

In therapy, remembering includes innumerable small interactions related to the trauma. The encounter with each one of them takes place from time to time, provided that other aspects of the abuse can be forgotten. When the child cannot think through all the parts as a whole and connect between the different aspects of the experience, we linger with her at each of its aspects separately without pressing her and without reminding her of the entire complexity.

Processing the various aspects of the experience is many times possible, though not in the specific context of the trauma. For example, becoming familiar with the sensation and the feeling that arise when I'm told to do something I don't feel like doing.

With respect to the body, it is likely that there will be preoccupation with a certain position, a certain theme of movement, and a certain organ, at a certain intensity. For example, with a patient who commands the therapist to lie down, sit, or stand, we will, together with him, try to find the words for the sensation and feeling of that experience. During the session, we can ponder with him how it feels when one is told to lie down and do something about which he has no freedom to choose? How does it feel to be able to give instructions like those to someone else? How does the other person receive this, and more? Alvarez describes therapy with a six-year-old girl who repeatedly tells her doll, 'lie down'! That's all. Nothing happened after that. Later on, there was preoccupation with pushing a finger into Plasticine, with no attempt to create anything out of the Plasticine. She made a mark in it and this gave her pleasure. In the next stage, aggression towards the male doll appeared and in parallel, improvement outside the therapy setting. Presented with these acts, the therapist emphasises what the girl feels in her body during the session itself, and what she feels that the doll feels. By processing the different aspects of the experience in the 'here and now', the therapist provides the child with emotional nutrition in digestible portions (in minimal doses, Strachey, 1934).

In addition, according to Alvarez, the therapist must differentiate between thought and action and thus help build a sense of an internalised object that is not vengeful, violent, and abusive. The therapist must listen not only to the child's statements but also to the confusion that may be reflected in the body, given the lack of distinction between phantasy and action. For example, with a child who is standing and trembling and threatens to stab the therapist, the therapist should not reflect the child's desire to stab (to harm) but being afraid to stab. In this way, the therapist helps construct secure relations and formulate an abuse-free aspect in the child's psyche.

The therapist should permit moments of forgetting. After we build trust in a non-abusive world, one must respect, for moments at a time, the child's need to leave the abuse outside of treatment and thought. In proper development, the latency stage enables this same respite from sexual stimulation. This respite is a goal of therapy. For example, at certain stages of therapy, a patient may be preoccupied with the flexibility of her body and in deriving pleasure from its strength and the physical control over her muscles. Those same positions can be interpreted as a reconstruction of erotic and sexual gestures but the therapist should express admiration of her abilities and not begin a discussion about physical intimacy and sex education which the girl is not dealing with at all during these moments. Ultimately, the therapist should create a space in which to remember and forget at the same time. Here, the goal is to create integration between memory and normal life. Alvarez describes a girl who was abused at age four. At the beginning of therapy, the movements of her body and her drawings were characterised by tension, contraction, and restlessness. After a lengthy period in treatment, the girl drew a lighthouse resembling a phallus, but the important thing in the drawing was the light pouring out of the lighthouse. Alvarez suggests that there is meaning in relating to the light in particular, as an internalisation of the therapist's concern and to thus allow the lighthouse to be just a lighthouse without attempting to confront the girl with the additional memories manifest in the drawing.

Memory and forgetting in Dance/Movement Therapy

In Dance/Movement Therapy (DMT), observation of the body is analogous to the sequence of free associations in speech. The therapist is not an expert in body language but observes the process – what is not there, what is there, transitions, changes, changing intensities, and ranges – while listening to the feelings and memories that arise from the movement. It is curiosity about the kinetics. Attention is paid to the form of the body; it evokes transference processes by which material discovered from the body slowly become psychic material that can be mentalised.

The attunement the therapist makes with her body to meet the needs of the patient creates a space to ponder and express embodied knowledge – knowledge with which there is no other way to be in contact. But, no less important than this, the attunement the therapist makes, not infrequently for the first time in the patient's life, invites internalisation of the experiences of a normative body, health, hopefulness, a safe relationship, of an object which gives meaning to experience. The therapist practises, together with the patient, safe body experiences. These 'new body experiences' of synchrony and adaptation in which the child is guarded and protected and not invaded are 'forgetting' and they open up a space for remembering, as well as of respite for the psyche and the body from a life governed exclusively by the traces of the trauma.

Therapy should begin from the experience of concepts the child is lacking: protection, justice, and treatment characterised by self-respect and self-esteem. This is the basis of the therapy. Likewise, the therapist should practise identifying and verbalising somatic experiences which are unconnected to the terrifying experience. That is, what cannot be said in words can be encountered by listening to the body's stories. What cannot be forgotten due to it being barricaded in the body can, perhaps, be diminished through internalising normative, pleasant, protected, and hopeful body-mind experiences, and an object that can provide it with meaning.

Since thought is made thinkable in a very slow and gradual process which cannot be hurried (Alvarez, 1992), placing the therapist in the position of an investigator attempting to reveal whether or not trauma occurred, can reconstruct an invasive experience. In this context, Yarom emphasises: 'In a case where a therapist suspects the possibility of his patient having been the victim of sexual trauma, the recommendation is not to concentrate on attempting to reconstruct memories but rather, to focus on the sense of confusion, vagueness and inbuilt ignorance which the patient or the therapist experiences and with which they imbue the therapeutic space' (p. 176).

I will illustrate using a vignette from the case study of Gal, aged nine. Gal underwent harsh sexual abuse from the age of five to seven. In the first stage of therapy, her body is entirely contracted, she barely uttered a word, and spent the time rocking herself on a physio ball as if she adopted it in order to sense the boundaries of her body and to attain some sense of calm. The therapist notes that any attempt to get closer to her was accompanied by Gal's muscles becoming rigid; when the therapist sat farther and her gaze was indirect, she combined this with making a sound so as to join the rhythm of the rocking, which allowed Gal deeper breaths and slower and more fluid movement. At one of the sessions, when Gal gets on top of the physio ball, she asked the therapist to 'watch over me' and when she approached, she moved wildly in a manner which left the therapist helpless and Gal in an unprotected place. The therapist took a ball, faced her, and reflected Gal's movement like a mirror. She searched for the size and intensity which would be precise in reflecting the stories being expressed out of her body. The meticulous joining slowly created a shared enjoyment.

When Gal's movement became faster, the therapist arranged pillows around herself and asked Gal if she would like to create protective buffers for herself. The therapist helped Gal to check how much space she needed for herself without feeling invaded or left alone. The movement opposite her was calming and provided a primal experience of connection to a mother who sees her and restores her to herself, as it were. This is the first and essential stage in treatment of sexual abuse with children.

After a number of weeks of treatment, Gal uses the ball as a starting point from where she checks out the room. At one of the sessions, she discerned a box full of balls and she came alive. She had a teasing look on her face and her eyes were frightened. She took a ball in her hand and said, 'I'll throw it at you'. In response, the therapist mirrored the noticeable fear in her gaze but not the aggressive elements: 'You're afraid that if you throw it, it will be so hard and I will get hurt'. The therapist steered her so that she could throw the ball at the wall in order to allow expression of her intensity, of the anger and rage, which only through an actual expression can begin to be told. The therapist asked Gal if the intensity of the throw accurately corresponded to the anger inside. Gal said no. She invited her to assign a number to the intensity of the throw and each time, to increase in intensity. This is how she listened to the story through the body and began to get to know the parts of her psyche while she was protected and safeguarded.

As seen in this chapter, therapy, particularly in childhood, in proximity to the trauma is essential. However, at every stage later on in life (adolescence, facing adult sexuality, entering into a relationship, parenthood, and old age), the intolerability of the abuse can emerge and once again demand a space for memory and solid ground upon which it is also possible to forget. For me, the poems of Yehuda Amichai (1998), an Israeli poet, amalgamate the thoughts woven through this chapter. In one poem, he writes: 'Their minds will remember so that I can rest', and in another, '... Sometimes the memory is the land ... and sometimes the memory is the sea which covers all ...' (p. 112). Like the body, the poem holds that which cannot be remembered and provides a bit of comfort and respite within the encounter with those primal horrors.

References

Alvarez, A. (1992). Child sexual abuse: The need to remember and the need to forget. In A. Alvarez, *Live company: Psychoanalytic psychotherapy with autistic, borderline, deprived and abused children* (pp. 151–163). London: Routledge.

Amichai, Y. (1998). *Open closed open*. New York: Schocken Publishing (Hebrew).

Bromberg, P. M. (1998). *Standing in spaces*. Hillsdale, NJ: The Analytic Press.

Gaitini, M. (2020). The unthinkable: Representation and the encounter with trauma. *The Psychoanalytic Review, 107*(6), 499–515.

Gurevich, H. (2010). The language of absence. *Sichot, 25*(1) 1–20. (Hebrew).

Hartmann, E. (1984). *The nightmare*. New York, NY: Basic Books.

Salcedo, D. (2007). http://www.tate.org.uk/modern/exhibitions/dorissalcedo/default.shtm

Strachey, J. (1934). The nature of the therapeutic action of psychoanalysis. *International Journal of Psycho-Analysis, 15*, 321–338.

Yarom, N. (2013). *Body dialects: Illuminating mental phenomena as expressed in the body*. Tel Aviv: Pardes (Hebrew).

Chapter 2

Diagnosis and Assessment of Sexual Abuse in Childhood Based on Bodily Expression

Einat Shuper Engelhard and Yana Sichel

Introduction

Frequently, when a suspicion of sexual abuse arises in therapy, the child's actions constitute the main channel for sharing the abuse. This chapter addresses the dynamic meanings of the body and its movements, and examines ways in which the existence of child sexual abuse can be discerned based on manifestations and expressions of the body. A case study is used to demonstrate and to propose insights relating to Dance/Movement Therapy (DMT) interventions needed at various stages of treatment.

In therapy with children, when a suspicion arises concerning sexual abuse, the treatment receives a jolt which pierces the therapist's body and heart. This chapter presents the therapy of a young girl, which was ongoing from the end of her primary school years to the middle of adolescence. Discussion of the case will delve into the role of the therapist's kinaesthetic attunement in situations where verbal discourse is not the bridge into the patient's psyche; it will address the dynamic meaning of body and movement and of situations where there is a diagnostic question as to whether sexual abuse took place.

Jenna begins treatment at 11 years of age. The official reason for the referral is social anxiety, though there also is a history of persistent enuresis, which enters into the picture as well. That is, functionally, the symptoms were avoidance and reduction, a freeze response when leaving the home. In the body, the symptoms express release and leakage, out of control, and the absence of holding.

At the first session, outside the treatment room, Jenna is glued to her mother and looks as if she is part of her and her body. The dynamic of their relations is reflected in her body, and her mother's close proximity calms and swallows her up at the same time. The therapist is witness to Jenna shrinking into herself as well as her avoidant behaviour but also to the oppositional force she displays which will, perhaps, serve her well as things progress.

She waits for permission to sit, does not lean against the back of the chair, her shoulders are slumped, her hands are clasped together, taut,

DOI: 10.4324/9781003309048-4

and contracted. The embodied object relations are expressed by passive internal holding, obvious effort, and difficulty relaxing, with only her toes touching the floor. She straightens up slightly, and makes intermittent eye contact only when the therapist sits down by her side. For her, secure attachment in her body occurs when communication is not face-to-face; she thus manages to sense enough calm to, at moments, create a body-to-body encounter.

Through her attempt to conceal her moving body and with clothing that is too big for her and blur her small body, she expresses a hope to be given over to the therapist and therapy: 'If only I could come here every day', she says and immediately begins to share the lyrics to songs she loves. Her thirst for permanent and continued holding can be felt. Thoughts of concealment and discovery will accompany the therapist throughout the treatment and there was a sense that only with distance from the sessions might there be an opening to come closer again in order to reveal what cannot be encountered and seen during therapy.

Initial self-presentation: Bounciness and repetitive movement

In the initial sessions, Jenna repeatedly recites lyrics from songs which, for her, are like a 'second skin' and create a self-holding envelope (Anzieu, 1985). In the body and in movement, the repetition of the same content for long periods of time is prominent with movement quality that is limited and fixed. Session after session, Jenna skips around while holding an imaginary teddy bear. This is her way of entering a relationship and of telling of herself. The therapist joins her in the body movements, signals to Jenna that she sees her and wants to get to know the sensation she experiences in her body and together, they leap around the room. The leaps symbolise the need for release and discharge. According to Kestenberg movement profile (Kestenberg-Amighi & Loman, 1999), the rhythm of the jumping enables the discharge of feeling of 'pleasure and excitement' through the homogenous use of all the body's organ as a single unit. This is a rhythm which expresses occupation with boundaries and blurring them. By jumping, the body seeks to enter into new spaces and is likely to symbolise a phantasy to blur internal and external, truth and fabrication, good and bad.

During this period, Jenna needs the therapist to join her in precise synchrony, to be 'together with her' in the movement. This is the primal holding, a merging in which there is no distinction between her and the therapist. They are together in body, with the same movement and the same effect. The repetition over time of the same narrow theme in movement can tell of how overwhelmed Jenna was when she began treatment. The therapist joining in her movement, and Jenna's body, slowly facilitate a change in movement and contact with additional psychic regions.

Chaos is revealed in the body – Separation in movement as a way to observe relations

After a lengthy period in treatment, the therapist proposes to Jenna that they move separately from one another. This is by means of a 'mirror game' in which each one suggests a movement and her partner joins her. The therapist invites an encounter with Jenna's spontaneous movement; these are free associations in movements which embody experience within a relationship. The therapist stands facing Jenna, waits for the movement to arrive and Jenna's body is all over the place without any gathering capability. Her movement reveals gaps between parts of her body, between the frozen centre and the turbulent and sloppy edges of her body. The therapist lends her body in the movement, like a mother who reflects herself back to her child so that the latter can get a sense of herself, and so as to support the experience of the 'going on being' – a physical motor experience in which organ follows organ in a sequence without interruption.

Alongside the therapist's efforts to attune to Jenna, however, she has difficulty following her. Her movement transitions are sharp and quick and do not allow an 'experience of togetherness'. Even when the therapist is leading them in a simple movement, Jenna has difficulty in organising her body and using the sensory surface the therapist offers her for the movement she is demonstrating with her own body. Jenna does not succeed in mimicking the therapist's movements and in making use of them in order to sense herself. The breakdown reflected in her body is on a very primal level.

In his writings on the autistic-contiguous experience, Ogden (2018) relates to an essential position in the development of personality in which the body is a central element of the entire psychic experience. According to him, an experience of feeling, with an emphasis on body form and rhythm, is the basis for the most fundamental system of infantile object relations. In the experience of feeling, Ogden sees a main means for creating psychological meaning and the basis for the experience of the self and object relations. In his view, formation of a coherent surface on which the self can develop is made possible through experience with external objects, usually by the process of imitation. These processes are a developmental platform for the creation of symbols.

Ogden provides an illustration from his treatment of a patient who for many years lived in a world devoid of meaning. The form initial contact with the patient took was imitating Ogden's stance, the tenor of his voice, and his every movement. The patient used Ogden's movements as a second skin or as a container inside which he tried, in a primitive manner, to feel alive. Another example of somatic mirroring can be found in Winnicott's writings (1965) where he describes how a therapist was able to communicate with a child patient by doing everything the child did. He would sit for a quarter hour without moving and then he would move his leg a little;

then she would move her foot. Winnicott notes that prior to this, the child was treated by a therapist who made clever interpretations and there was progress to a certain extent, but in his reading of the situation, what gave the push to the therapy was the movement communication in which the previous analyst engaged.

As mentioned, in the initial meetings with Jenna, even primal and primitive experiences of joining in a movement and imitation were not possible. Jenna's body tells of the sense of failure and the loneliness she feels in relations.

The biting rhythm – Marking body boundaries and separation

The assumption in DMT is that physical positions and spontaneous expressions of movement constitute body-mind mechanisms of the muscle and respiratory envelope. With his body, the patient tells us 'this is how I can manage in the world, only in this way is it possible'. By joining in with the patient's movement, precisely as needed, expanding or contracting the movement, varying the beat, the intensity, and its size in the space, the therapist listens and is intrigued by the patient's body-mind experience (Shuper Engelhard, 2018). In treating Jenna, the therapist notices that the imaginary teddy bear with which Jenna dances falls down and Jenna points an accusatory finger at him during the movement, which becomes dramatic and intensifies. In response, the therapist slightly increases the intensity of the movement as if saying to Jenna, 'it's ok to get angry, to be in pain, to feel the intensity of your body'.

Gradually, the dance changes and they are together in anger, stamping their feet. Through the body, the therapist gives legitimacy to the experience of shoving and separation. The foot stamping expresses the biting rhythm which, in the developmental process, appears along with the eruption of the first teeth and allows the infant an experience of separation from the mother's body. It is a sharp movement at low intensity which enables, with a tap on the body, for example, an experience of body boundaries (for more on rhythms, see Kestenberg-Amighi & Loman, 1999).

Shared breathing – Providing resources for cohesion in the face of bodily tension and discomfort

During the second year of treatment, Jenna deals with content about doctors and patients. The content repeats itself and by listening to its rhythms, it is possible to identify interruptions and sharp and rapid transitions. In transference processes, the therapist feels tension in her body and discomfort; the content is not ultimately expressed and materialised, and there is the sense of experience slipping through one's fingers every time and not being fully told. Like a nightmare which returns again and again, the play in the room arouses fear without the possibility of discharging it or defending against it.

Following this experience, at the end of the session the therapist invites Jenna to an experience of physical cohesion, an invitation to pay attention to breathing, inhalation, and exhalation. She guides Jenna to attend to the soles of her feet supported by the floor and to relate to three senses in her body. Jenna, however, does not succeed in telling of her physical experience in words, in identifying her feelings and expressing them. The therapist lends herself to Jenna and demonstrates: 'a tingling in my foot', 'an itch in my ear', and Jenna repeats the therapist's feelings as if they were her own. Jenna needs the therapist in order to be attentive to her own physical feelings. That is, now she is already able to use the therapist's physical skin in order to get a sense of herself, however, without a clear separation between the bodily experiences of each.

Movement without emotional expression – Expanding movement as a bridge to making contact with emotional experience

Treatment continues and there is much movement, play, and use of imagination in the room but they are detached from emotion. There is a sense that Jenna's movement is a cover for terrifying regions in her psyche. 'Let's dance together with scarves' the therapist proposes, with the desire to summon emotional expression of internal experience by expressing new movement qualities. The therapist actively proposes switching hands, directions, and different heights. Jenna cooperates and enjoys herself.

The movement stimulus is intended to arouse somatic associations and to slowly try to extract body-mind experiences from the depths. At this stage, Jenna's remarks following the movement are concrete: yellow is the feeling of the sun, blue is the feeling of a stormy sea. This is her way of beginning to denote experience and the words she chooses emphasise the extent of the paucity and narrowness of her emotional language.

The therapist attempts to arouse in Jenna emotional movement, movement with no formative, aesthetic, or performative intent. Aesthetic movement frequently characterises the movement of patients at the beginning of the therapeutic relationship. Movement out of attentiveness to one's inner world is possible only after gaining trust. This kind of movement is associated with loosening the awareness of time and reality and with primal thought processes (Shuper Engelhard, 2017).

Encountering non-verbal experiences – An invitation to tell with the body

Object relations theories and later on, relational and intersubjective theories emphasise the importance of physical and mental holding and the attunement of the mother's body to the infant's body, which constitutes the infrastructure for creating a body-mind envelope in infancy. These processes are demonstrated in Jenna's treatment.

In the hallway, before entering the session, the therapist discerns that Jenna's eyes are red. Her mother says: 'She's hot, is there an air conditioner in the room'?

In the session, Jenna tells of the incident, in which she cried, was tense, and trembled. 'I didn't understand if it was because I was cold or afraid'. The therapist explains to her how to identify and understand the body's feelings: 'Fear serves us and protects us. It helps us understand that we need to be careful'. Jenna looks at the therapist as if she were swallowing her words. Jenna needs holding that has no fear of the search for her subjectivity, a search which requires the therapist's attunement and calm in the face of uncertainty. Only through searching will it be possible to get in touch with the source of her body's trembling. It is a search for Jenna's needs, feelings, and emotions in the aim of helping her learn to identify and name the feelings and emotions in her body.

In another session, the therapist sensed that Jenna was experiencing discomfort in her body and that her smile was forced and told of worry. She asks her about the experience at home but Jenna pushes away any possibility of conversation. She is not capable of speaking 'about', her body contracts and she withdraws. According to Levine (2012), a psychoanalyst who discusses primal mental states, in cases where words do not lead to an encounter with psychic stories, it is the motoric acts that are unavoidable and essential in order to get in touch with the patient's inner world. Later on in the session, the therapist asks Jenna how she feels with her friends, but this time she suggests that she demonstrate with her body. Jenna cooperates. With her body she is able to have discussions with the therapist. She stands with her back to the wall and does not move. In order to sense the feeling together with her, the therapist stands with her and for moments, the two stand still. The therapist is intrigued by the experience, invites Jenna to name the feelings. She asks about the feeling in her limbs and Jenna answers: 'My hands and feet want to play and my eyes become tired just from looking'. Again, a split between the parts of the body and desires and the therapist is filled with sadness. With an invitation to movement, the therapist, together with Jenna, searches for what the body knows how to tell. Through the body and the movement, it is possible to be in touch with the feelings and emotions, and together think through psychic regions that are not yet recorded in the mind.

Reinforcement for this way of working is found in neuropsychological studies that show that a single traumatic event is sufficient for it to be recorded in the amygdala forever; its record in the primitive regions will be tied to smell, sound, touch, 'a story without a story' (Cassorla, 2013). Therefore, under the right conditions, the sensory stimulation of the 'here and now' leads to an encounter with raw psychic elements. Thus, in the aim of creating or reinforcing the representation ability, during the course of therapy, we are called upon to relive moments in which the senses were at the centre of experience, and to repeat the primitive process of indwelling of the psyche in the soma. In DMT, the kinaesthetic sense, the sensation of the muscles, joints, limbs, and tendons during movement and the various body positions as well as absorbing stimuli such as heat, pain, and form through the skin are central in the analytical movement experience (Shuper Engelhard, 2018).

Gurevich (2015) emphasises that in analysis there is a tendency to repeat psychic states that have not been represented. In her view, if the therapist understands that this is the gist of the matter, his goal will be to actually and actively revive the 'thing' that has not undergone mentalisation and which is expressed through action. In this way, the not-represented and erased can be constructed, and the functions which the earlier environment did not manage to complete, can be completed.

In psychic regions which have not yet been processed, the suggestion to treat using body movement allows a somatic search of experiences. Through movement of the body, the patient experiences shards of somatic sensations. Processing them in the therapeutic relationship is the way out of wallowing in them (Shuper Engelhard, 2018). Levine (2012) suggests that in regions that cannot be represented, the therapist's psyche must be active, to build the 'here and now' through mirroring the sequence of events in the session and the emotion which the interaction gave rise to, and to remind the patient of what was said, felt, or happened just a moment ago. The therapist actively helps the patient transfer the experience from action to thought, without it being erased.

Shuper Engelhard (2018) explains how the movement assists in the process of turning the experience into a representation: DMT proposes a preliminary stage in which an invitation to movement summons a somatic search of unconscious experiences which, up to now, were not possible to reach through verbal discussion alone; thus, its construction begins with '"*somatic figurability*"' (this concept corresponds to the concept of psychic figurability which serves Botella and Botella (2005) in describing the initial representational work of assigning form to what, until now, evaded representation). That is, the rhythm, space, weight, directionality and intensity of the kinaesthetic experience embodied in the body. This is reflected in the breathing, position of the organs, the range of movement and its characteristics, in muscular tension, heartbeat, physical stance, and in the experience of physical stability or its absence, and more' (p. 6).

Shuper Engelhard (2018) describes the type of intervention required in such situations:

> The psychic continua are experienced in the "here and now" of the analytical relationships in the body of the analyst and the body of the patient. The therapist helps the patient to think the experience

in the body by inviting movement and observing it. Later on, joining in with aspects of the movement as a whole or with some parts of it, makes it possible to give form to something that previously was only marginally represented.

(p. 12)

Between disconnection and respite and between passivity and intensity

In the third year of treatment, Jenna's body changes quickly and looks as if it is 'too big on her'. When she walks her entire body moves, the arms are all over, the pelvis moves from side to side. This same girl who tried to be swallowed up and disappear now conveys an exposed presence. Her gait is a heavy weight and passive, her legs are thrown about as if moving on their own. Like a rag doll, with no gathering and holding, which are all the more conspicuous in light of her choice of either very tight or very large clothing, always in pinks.

Jenna dives into another imaginary game, she builds infinite worlds in the room, more and more buildings and cities, in infinite numbers and only the journey between them allows for a moment of rest. In the room there is chaos, and the game has a manic quality. It is a rapid game, without boundaries, rocky, everything changes, threatens, and grows all the time. The therapist feels exhaustion, confusion, and purposelessness. Thieves threaten to invade and destroy everything and Jenna wires the room with security cameras. The therapist emphasises: 'There are secrets and things hidden from sight which require safeguarding and security'.

At the end of these sessions, in order to gather Jenna, the therapist invites her to come to the mats so she can scan her body's organs. The therapist joins her for movement on the mat in order 'to be with her in the experience', this time lying horizontally alongside each other, and not standing vertically as in the first year of treatment. The therapist lends her body, tries to concentrate on breathing, guides Jenna to pay attention to thoughts, feelings, emotions which arise and what they are, and to return her attention to inhalation and exhalation. Like a mother, the therapist teaches Jenna to 'think her body'.

Using joint breathing as a way to produce emotional integration and to become aware of a snippet of psychic reality which the patient cannot tell about in words, is mentioned in Winnicott's writings. Winnicott (1949) observes the body and reacts with movements of his own body. For example, he observes the changes in this patient's breathing (which, in his view, should be meticulously monitored) and the body's muscle contractions (which, he notes, should be experienced anew and in this way, recalled). In one case, he describes a 47-year-old female patient. In the treatment sessions, Winnicott 'was holding her and keeping a continuity by his own breathing', and by listening and observing the movements of the patient's belly as she breathed.

Gradually, Jenna's reflective ability develops. She can now discern her own feelings and say: 'My right hand is tired', 'a feeling of cold in my hands'. At another session she relates: 'Dad made noise with his shoes and it gave me goose bumps all over my body and I cried'. Jenna tells of experience in her body which takes place within a relationship and of the emotion aroused within her as a result of the feeling. The new language she is developing in treatment enables her to identify emotion and to express herself.

Physical-emotional memory breaks through

The therapist is surprised to discover that Jenna sleeps with her father and mother in the same bed – a fact told to the therapist in an offhand manner. Lying down beside the therapist on the mat leads Jenna to declare: 'I couldn't sleep, my brain sleeps but my stomach and my head don't'. Jenna was perhaps relating that it is possible for thoughts to be split from the body, not to think but to experience it in the body. 'It's hard for me to fall asleep at night'. She relates that it is difficult for her to relax her body and for the first time, speaks of an unpleasant touch which morning does away with. 'I'm afraid of the dark, I cover myself up with my blanket and imagine that it's already morning and no one is touching me'. This sentence raises questions for the therapist and connects to images from sessions where at times, Jenna would touch her genitals and sniff her fingers, or she would scratch her behind and sniff. Exposed, defenceless, she tells of disconnection and checks the kind of content that can be expressed in therapy. The therapist tries to encourage her to share, to hear more from her about this experience but she receives no response. Jenna signals that this is an area that is off-limits and which has no words.

Giving legitimacy to expressions of fear, power, and intensity

In the following sessions, a game with a new quality begins. Jenna assigns the therapist the role of the good protector and she has the role of tyrant. Entrance to the game is through an imaginary fairy tale door, each time using a different movement. There is variation in the body and a clear border between imagination and reality. Many sessions begin with the characters sleeping and then in the dark, the evil character is involved in hiding, lying, and concealment. In a process of projective identification, the therapist feels tiredness during the game. At first she hides it and swallows her yawns because she feels uncomfortable about it but later on, she allows the fatigue a place and does not try to cover up: 'Oh, someone is trying to put me to sleep'. Jenna answers: 'There are things that need to be hidden'. In the game there are secrets which Jenna assures 'will be revealed in time', and the therapist is left frightened and defenceless.

Jenna enthusiastically enters the roles of the different characters, and allows herself to move in the entire space and to switch between voices, tones, and intensities. The tone is so different from her regular voice, which is weak and embarrassed. She begins to take up space, to discover and to be discovered, to express aggressive content and to speak more emotion. Good characters become evil in an instant. In slow motion, Jenna removes the mask from the good character (in contrast with her rapid movements in the manic game), bares her teeth, and rolls her eyes with a wicked laugh. The therapist feels her heart beating and gives voice to the feeling: 'I'm afraid'. And then Jenna goes to the lavatory. Jenna feels her body and her digestive system and seeks a place for privacy, unlike the pee which flows uncontrolled in the bed.

In the process of projective identification, the therapist partially experiences the patient's feelings in his or her own body, falls into a reverie in their regard, and reflects these feelings back to the patient in a form that can be more readily thought (Bion, 1970). The therapist dreaming the physical sensations implanted into his or her being recreates the primal communication between the mother and infant prior to the advent of speech, when all the infant had the senses and the body. In the process of reverie, the therapist connects between sensation, emotion, and memory and in this manner, concrete physical sensations become symbolic and hold emotional significance. These processes, when they are repeatedly experienced, constitute the infrastructure for reflectivity.

Jenna's body changes along with the characters. The good characters skip around the room with light movements, and the evil characters whose walk is robot-like. Experimentation enables Jenna to feel different qualities in herself and they summon, in her movement, a new hue, gathered, directly focused, and in a slower rhythm. The therapist proposes a freeze intervention for the game. The cessation constitutes a respite and time to practise lingering in and contemplating the experience, in contrast to the anesthetising and disconnecting sleep which appeared at the beginning. In the game, Jenna practises a feeling of power and expression of anger and intensity. Treatment provides a space, which strengthens the liveliness in her psyche in contrast with the fatigue and helplessness. In this stage as well, as opposed to entering the game, exiting it is difficult for Jenna. She remains in character even when the game ends and is frustrated by the transition from the play space to reality.

Jenna internalises the ability to use her body for the purpose of organising psychic experience. In the game, she teaches the protector witchcraft with which to fight shyness: she stands straight and drums on her body. The therapist has trouble following her; her movements are all over the place and rapid. This time, however, unlike in the mirror game in the initial sessions, she knows that Jenna is open to hearing her because her explanation is needed so that the therapist can be with her in the game. 'One minute, I didn't understand', the therapist asks her to slow down and repeat the movement. In the game, the therapist invites her to pay attention to her body, to know her movement and herself. The therapist's listening to the psychic story told by the body enables development of Jenna's experience of herself and the deepening of the feeling of ownership of her emotional experiences.

The therapist's attunement to the changes in position of Jenna's body, to the distance of the parts from the centre of the body, to intensity, to directionality, to speed of movement point her attention to 'beta elements' of the psyche, sensory-somatic qualities. Lingering there summons Jenna to a shared pre-verbal experience. The assumption in DMT is that the sensory experience will facilitate, eventually, an 'alpha process', transforming the somatic experience into thoughts. Thus, instead of acting in an unconscious manner, the therapist invites Jenna to a somatic experience in which the main communication takes place in the body-mind theatres.

In later sessions, when the therapist signals that the session must end, Jenna moves frenetically and begins to drum on herself. Here, the drumming serves her so that she is able to feel the boundaries of her body, as a substitute for the 'envelope' of the imaginary play. The therapist joins in the shared drumming and they can take turns and change rhythms. The drumming is now her power and emotional regulation and communication with the therapist. Now, the fact that the game is over is clear; the therapist and Jenna leave through the fairy tale door, shake their bodies, drum on them, and Jenna signals who was who in the game and who they are now, a distinction enabled by the sense of the body's boundaries. When the therapist guides Jenna to place a hand on her heart and a hand on her abdomen to pay attention to her breathing and heartbeats, Jenna is frightened and asks: 'It's beating fast, is that ok?' Jenna takes interest in her body and a discussion develops about the body and feelings. Together it is possible to give meaning to feelings.

All through Jenna's treatment, there were moments of stimulation, disconnection, and alertness. Jenna expresses interest in playing with the inflatable bobo doll; she lies down on it and spreads herself out on it, sometimes wraps her legs around it. The therapist is witness to her search for sensation in the whole of the front of her body, her chest, and internal organs which seek contact with objects in the room, while at the same time, Jenna describes a fear of coughing, blowing her nose, and touching her body. She lies on the pouffe while hugging it with her arms and legs. At times, she sits facing the therapist with her legs spread apart, with her underpants exposed, inadvertently. The therapist feels uncomfortable. Doubts arise: is this childish behaviour or a cry for help? In later sessions, her clothes are stained and Jenna often bunches her wide blouse in between her legs, at times holds the pouffe between her legs, and moves around uncomfortably in her chair.

Jenna tells stories with her body and expresses, at the beginning of treatment, massive difficulties in emotional thinking, detachment from her body, and a lack of control over her body. Problems in thinking, including difficulty contemplating, concretising, difficulty remembering oneself and thinking about oneself, a detached perception of reality and deficiency in attributing meaning. The disconnection from the body includes dissociated states, disconnection from bodily sensations, over-investment in or lack of acceptance of the body, doubts about the body, limitation of motion, and a sense of lack of ownership, understanding or control over the body: debilitation, neglect, and more. The assumption in DMT is that movement enables psychological aspects to be connected to one another: thought, perception, symbolic processing of experience to somatic and kinaesthetic experience.

In the case study presented, it is not known whether Jenna was a victim of sexual abuse but the diagnostic question regarding danger and protection certainly comes up. Young children who experience sexual trauma, not only that the trauma prevents reflective thinking, at times like with Jenna, but that reflective abilities never matured in the first place. That is to say, many times the abused child does not yet know how to differentiate between 'I' and 'you' (to understand that someone did this to me and I felt that he is not allowed to). At times, the abused child does not yet know how to differentiate between imagination and reality, between thought and action, how to identify a feeling or emotion and name it.

According to Alvarez (1992), when trauma takes place at very young ages and cannot be treated close to the time of its occurrence, and the child is not familiar with the healthy circumstances of non-abuse, impairment of developmental processes will be seen and a disparity between chronological age and mental age. The symptoms are likely to manifest in:

- Weaning difficulties, somatic pains
- Cognitive 'holes', disruption of memory, attention, and learning functions
- Regulation and executive function difficulties
- Difficulty in enjoying learning, creative activities, and play
- Obsessive, repetitive, and concrete activities
- Restless movement

Many times, in treatment, before the child is able to remember the trauma, the faculty of thinking must be developed. The child must be capable of making the connection between thought, emotion, and action, to identify and verbalise even those somatic experiences not related to the trauma. Later on, the trauma should be represented through sensory experiences, that is, the closest thing to the actual, that very experience which, due to the dissociative mechanism, cannot be mentalised using language which has rules and order. Memories told by the body must be contained by the therapist for long periods of time without rushing to confront the patient with them (Joseph, 1978). Situations in which the child, in a projective identification process, deposits intolerable experiences with the therapist requires the therapist to enable the child to investigate the experience in a safe and more tolerable context (Alvarez, 1992). Dramatising the trauma and reconstructing it in the body can appear as an attempt to cast the therapist as a victim or aggressor, exactly as in the tyrant game in Jenna's treatment. In such situations, the therapist should reflect the emotional experience of each one of the partners to the 'here and now' in order to practise reflective, emotional discussion.

With respect to perverted behaviour, the therapist should protect the child on the concrete level and contain the psychic materials in a better way than the child himself is capable of – the therapist serves as a self-object to feel and speak the fear, the insult, the rage which that perverted behaviour arouses. Occasionally, a long period of time passes until the experience becomes less overwhelming and can be digested. The representation is a developmental achievement which is made possible by the presence of an attuned mother who adapts to the body and turns the existence of nothingness into a space to dream and fantasise. In DMT, mirroring and naming somatic and kinaesthetic aspects in the attuned relationship support construction of a reflective function which is, in principle, the ability to give meaning in the psyche to somatic experiences. Thereafter, slowly, a space is created for memory of the unthinkable.

Jenna's treatment presents a number of warning signs expressed in the body:

- Unconscious touching of the body
- Repetitiveness of content
- Lack of organisation in movement
- Fatigue and detachment
- Difficulty entering and exiting imaginary play
- Disconnection between body parts and a misdirected search for calm

From the therapist's interventions, we learn about the uniqueness of bodily interventions in DMT:

- Joining the movement of the patient as a means of creating trust and a primal connection
- Engaging in the mirror game to become familiar with spontaneous expressions of movement in relations

- Engaging in the freeze game as an invitation to linger in an emotional experience
- Inviting the patient to tell an emotional experience with the body
- Invitation to expand and vary movement as a means of expressing an emotional experience
- Creating a space to express chaos, fear, and intensity along with practising relaxation
- Practising sensing the body's boundaries to achieve regulation and an experience of protection in the relationship
- The therapist's encouragement to increase or decrease the intensity of movement as a means of being exposed to various psychic phenomena
- Expanding the movement with the use of an accessory
- Verbalising body experiences, joining in and investigating them

As Jenna's treatment continues, the arousal of the body must be considered. The continuing bed-wetting must enter the therapeutic discussion in order to open another space to be with Jenna and the experiences in her psyche. It is possible that such adjustment on the part of the therapist will be possible through projective work 'close to the experience', with objects spilling about the room, attention to changing body temperature, warmth contrasted with cold, a sense of leakage and release in contrast to control and holding, etc. Throughout the intervention, the invitation to body-mind integration should be continued while addressing the sequence of experiences in the session, discerning the narratives which take place in the 'here and now', and paying attention to action which arouses emotion, image and movement.

According to Winnicott (1971), in play, intrapsychic processes are actually represented. This is an exciting, fragile, and vulnerable experience, which occurs as a result of the magic within the intimacy, in relations that are worthy of trust. Above all, the trust and safety provided to Jenna in treatment are the protection and the envelope essential in order to flourish from unprotected experiences towards a sense of protection and pleasure in the psyche and the body, and in relationships with her environment.

References

Alvarez, A. (ed.). (1992). Child sexual abuse: The need to remember and the need to forget. In *Live company: Psychoanalytic psychotherapy with autistic, borderline, deprived and abused children* (pp. 151–163). London: Routledge.

Anzieu, D. (1985). *The skin ego*. Tel Aviv: Tola'at Sfarim (Hebrew translation).

Bion, W. R. (1970). *Attention and interpretation*. London: Tavistock Pub.

Botella, C., & Botella, S. (2005). *The work of psychic figurability: Mental states without representation*. Hove; New York, NY: Brunner Routledge.

Cassorla, R. (2013). Reflections on non-dreams-for-two, enactment and the analyst's implicit alpha function. In H. Levine & L. Brown (Eds.), *Growth and turbulence in the container/contained*. Hove; New York, NY: Brunner Routledge.

Gurevich, H. (May, 2015). Discussion at lecture by Dr. Howard Levine, 'Clinical implications of unrepresented states: Erasure, discourse and construction'. Lecture presented at 'Absence of mental representation – Theoretical and clinical aspects'. Tel Aviv: Tel Aviv University (Hebrew).

Joseph, B. (1978). Different types of anxiety and their handling in the analytic situation. *International Journal of Psychoanalysis*, *59*, 223–228.

Kestenberg-Amighi, J., & Loman, S. (1999). Interpreting a KMP of Carlos, a three-and-one-half-year-old boy: An illustrative case. In J. Kestenberg-Amighi, S. Loman, & P. Lewis (Eds.), *The meaning of movement: Developmental and clinical perspectives of the Kestenberg movement profile* (pp. 291–308). New York, NY: Brunner Routledge.

Levine, H. B. (2012). The colourless canvas: Representation, therapeutic action and the creation of mind. *International Journal of Psychoanalysis*, *93*, 607–629.

Ogden, T. H. (2018). *The primitive edge of experience*. New York, NY: Brunner Routledge.

Shuper Engelhard, E. (2017). Body and movement in dynamic psychotherapy: Reflections on talking and movement therapies. *Body, Movement and Dance in Psychotherapy*, *12*(2), 98–110.

Shuper Engelhard, E. (2018). Somatic mirroring: Psychotherapeutic treatment of mental states without representation. *Body, Movement and Dance in Psychotherapy*, *13*(1), 4–16. https://doi.org/10.1080/17432979.2017.1408685

Winnicott, D. W. (1949), Mind and its relation to the psyche-soma. In: *Through pediatrics to psycho-analysis*. New York, NY: Basic Books.

Winnicott, D. W. (1965). Letter to Michael Fordham, 15 July 1965. In F. R. Rondan (Ed.), *The spontaneous gesture: Selected letters of D. W. Winnicott* (pp. 150–151). Cambridge, MA: Harvard University Press.

Winnicott, D. W. (1971). *Playing and reality*. Tel Aviv: Am Oved (Hebrew translation).

Dance/Movement Therapy with Adolescents

Dance/Movement Therapy
with Adolescents

Chapter 3

From the Freeze Response to Free Flow in Dance Movement Therapy with Sexually Abused Adolescent Girls

Orna Drori

Introduction

This chapter discusses the 'thawing' of frozen movement-cognitive-emotional processes using Dance Movement Therapy (DMT) with sexually abused adolescent girls. The first part describes socio-cultural-gender characteristics in the transition process from childhood to adolescence. These affect the movement, consciousness, and emotional changes in young girls and even more so, in teenage girls who were sexually abused. The second part delves into the phenomenon of the freeze response as a common physical-survival reaction of the body which is of crucial importance in the formation of complex post-traumatic stress disorder (CPTSD). The 'secret' is another element associated with sexual abuse, discussed in the chapter. The implications that keeping the secret have for the adolescent girl and the journey to its discovery are described. The chapter presents therapeutic elements that are basic and essential to the healing process in adolescence. Case studies illustrate the ways DMT employs movement, thought, and emotional processes to aid in the thawing of the freeze response and in moving towards free flow.

Oftentimes, the movement of adolescent girls is characterised by freezing, introversion, diminishment, shame, embarrassment, restraint, lack of confidence, and weakness (Elior, 2010), a way of being that can be called 'near-self experience'. Unlike adolescent girls, during the latency period, younger girls whose development is normal are generally girls with vitality. They appear self-confident, strong, fully present, move freely, that is, they engage in flowing movement in which the action of their muscles is harmonious. In her writings on Laban and Lawrence's theory of movement analysis (1947), Dell (1970) notes that free-flowing movement is linked to holding and release of emotions and urges. That is to say, the more fluid and harmonious a person's movement is, and a minimum of muscle exertion is invested in execution, the more adaptively it is possible to express inner feelings, thoughts, and urges. Consistent with this, latency-age girls who generally tend to move in a free-flowing manner appear to be more

DOI: 10.4324/9781003309048-6

emotionally connected to themselves and less embarrassed by surrounding society. Their presence may be described as a presence synchronous with the self, settled within it and flowing from it.

'Throwing like a girl'

In 1980, the political philosopher, I.M. Young, whose work concerns the essence of justice and the social differences between men and women, published an article titled, 'Throwing like a Girl', in which she addressed feminine movement and body experience as part of social existence. Unlike other philosophers before her, Young grasped the difference in development between the sexes as gender differences. That is to say, as those which emerge from socialisation processes and not as linked only to the physical differences between the sexes. Young claimed that the more the young girl internalises her feminine status, the more she adopts vulnerable body behaviour and less mobility in the public space. Teenage girls in the West grow up in a society based on male-patriarchal oppression and they thus learn how not to use full movement and spatial potential available to them (Young, 1980). More recent studies show that even currently, adolescent girls tend to internalise the male perspective with respect to their bodies and relate to them as a sexual object (Weinberg & Tamir, 2017, 2017). In the treatment of adolescent girls who are victims of sexual abuse, the approach in emotion-focused therapy is to relate to the girl, first and foremost, as a subject. That is, as a unique being who suffered sexual assault as a personal and private experience. At the same time, continuing Young's socio-cultural thinking, when we approach treatment of sexual abuse in therapy, it is important to relate to it as a phenomenon that exists in a socio-cultural-genderal context as well.

Adolescent girls are at an essential stage of building their personal-feminine identity and therefore, as part of therapy it should be explained and even 'taught', that they are not alone … meaning that there are more women and men who have experience sexual abuse and that an assault of this type has a broader socio-cultural-genderal context. Ziv (2012) expands on the socio-cultural conception with respect to sexual trauma and defines it as a private case of an 'insidious trauma' – a phenomenon which has meaning in the intra-psychic structure and in the 'political' structure as well.

Another significant aspect connected both to the maturation process and to sexual assault is the circular effect of assault to the body. The body-mind circular movement occurs thusly, the sexual assault experienced concretely in the body (penetration, unwanted external touch, inappropriate proximity) continues to exist and to be replayed in bodily symptoms (changes in body posture, eating habits and body weight, sleeping difficulties, degree of preoccupation with aesthetics and hygiene). The main purpose of therapy is to facilitate a mental transformation of the bodily symptoms and to bestow emotional and cognitive meaning to the bodily experience. This process is highly reminiscent of Bion's concept of *reverie*, in which raw beta particles, that is, wordless sensory and physical experiences, become, via a transformative process of mentalisation by another, alpha particles, which hold understanding and meaning. In the work of therapy with sexually abused adolescent girls, the dynamic circular process from the body to the mind and back again has great significance for understanding and processing the trauma.

The sexual assault impacts bodily processes, the sensory regulation systems, mobility, somatic phenomena, and emotional and mental processes, which take place during adolescence. In general, an adolescent girl left without parental response appropriate to her maturation processes may develop a behavioural mechanism of physicality, that is, increased and maladaptive preoccupation with the body and external appearance. Likewise, she may adopt an intellectual outlook concerning her body and movement and detach herself from her basic needs. Another coping pattern which may appear is a complete split between body and mind in which the body is experienced as foreign to the self (Shuper Engelhard, 2014). All these tendencies are exacerbated and intensify in a situation where a secret is continually kept and the sexual abuse the teenage girl underwent is concealed.

In DMT, the disconnection from the body can be expressed in diverse ways: in constricting the movement, that is, in minimising the range of the movement, in disconnection between body organs and/or body parts (head as opposed to the rest of the body, upper and lower parts separated at the pelvis), in general lack of motivation to move and/or to relate to the body and difficulty in moving, the source of which is in the freeze response. Following the polyvagal theory (Porges, 2011), I will expand upon detachment from the body as a type of freeze. According to Porges, freezing is a phenomenon that expresses mental and physical detachment which, in extreme situations, leads to a complete freeze of movement in space, to the point of somatic freezing of the body and mental detachment from it and from the situation. Dissociative detachment occurs as a result of the combination of a sense of threat and helplessness. That is, interpretation of the situation as unsafe, as an attack with no possibility of escape. This interpretation immediately arouses the primitive dorsal-vagal nerve, thus producing an extreme deceleration in heart rate and respiration and a reduction in the amount of oxygen supplied to the body. An adaptive fight/flight movement response is delayed and freezing occurs. At times, the heart rate slows to the point of fainting and/or feigning death (Porges), phenomena which are common in the therapy room when dealing with sexual trauma. For a teenage girl who experienced sexual abuse – it is highly likely that the treatment room in general, and the DMT treatment room in particular, will initially represent for her – consciously or unconsciously, a trigger for the threatening situation of assault. The therapeutic situation will be interpreted as threatening, whether because of its concern with the body or due to therapy being an intimate encounter between two people, with no other witness, just like the assault. From the young girl's perspective, a freeze response would be a survival tactic familiar from similar situations in the past, and an automatic one.

Therapy and recovery from cases such as these will occur as a result of a deep and long-term process in a safe and protected therapeutic relationship based on trust and an approach attuned to the body and to movement. In such an environment, the freeze response can undergo mentalisation processes and take on meaning and will not endure as a physical act alone. At times, it will be possible to see change in the attributes of movement, thawing and use of free flow. Below, a case description presents minimal movement intervention at the beginning of a relationship, which assists with relaxation and thawing the flow of the body and mind's movement (free flow).

Shir

Shir came to therapy at age 12. A child-adolescent. Skinny, a 'young bird' kind of look. Huge, beautiful eyes and a mane of hair. The reason for the referral was a sexual assault by a boy her age which, when it was discovered, exposed an earlier layer of ongoing abuse during childhood by a family member. During therapy, she was assaulted several times by boys her age. Shir was referred to me in order to try movement as a kind of therapy that would be 'a little different'. Her parents said that she loves to dance and therefore they thought that DMT would be able to engage her in the process.

Shir agreed to come to therapy and during the initial sessions she also agreed to move. It is not clear whether this was of her own free will or a decision which arose from her need to be obliging towards her parents/ me. Already in the first session, I suggested that she engage in movement. Apparently, I also felt obligated to the DMT 'label'. We started with a warmup. I asked whether she would like us to move in turns – once me, once her, but Shir preferred only to 'do what you do' and not to initiate her own original movement. Her movement was small and limited. The movements were not fully realised, 'until the end', and it seemed as if she was 'marking' the movement and not moving so as to completely follow through with it. In parallel, I noticed a contraction and rigidity in her neck. Something there appeared stuck, frozen, not flowing. Shir cracked her neck and said: 'Since Mum took me to the chiropractor who cracked me there, it hurts'. This led me to understand that treatment was, for her, a painful thing. At the end of the warmup, she said that in any case, she prefers hip-hop dance. I invited her to show me but very quickly, she became tired out, embarrassed. At the end of the session, she responded to relaxation, relishing the opportunity to lie down and rest. I was with her, understanding how much tension there was in her spare body.

In the second session, Shir told me that her entire body was cramped and she did not want to engage in movement. I understood that she felt somewhat freer about not pleasing others and capable of declaring a small 'no', and was perhaps hinting to me that the body work of the previous session was too direct for her. She laughed a lot, the laugh too – its unconscious purpose was to release inner tension. We worked on relaxation and on stretching her cramped muscles. Shir said it was relaxing. She responded and yielded to it, especially to massage with the ball. The contact with the body enabled her to tell me about the separation from her new boyfriend: 'He said that he'll think about it for a week and then give me an answer and I said to him: Haha … you think I'm going to wait a week for you?! Then I broke up with him'. I gave her positive reinforcement for taking control, but also said that in any case, it is hurtful when someone does not want to be in a relationship with us. Shir was detached from the emotional aspect.

In the third session, her movement was larger and more free-flowing. A flow of air and movement was apparent in the upper part of her body. In contrast, her knees were still rigid. At her own initiative, she switched to a juggling game – enjoyed it and was challenged. She didn't give up. It was hard and frustrating and the ball fell again and again but she fought, was not tense, and kept on picking up the balls. Shir is very critical of herself but she managed to say: 'I didn't know that about myself, that I don't give up'.

Already in these initial sessions, it was possible to discern that movement and attention to the somatic experience, in an immediate manner, enabled her to thaw a little of the freeze and to connect somewhat more to herself and her environment. The warmup, the stretches, the relaxation, and playing with the ball drew Shir's attention towards herself in a way that she was able to sense her body and afterwards, to feel her soul: What pains her? What is pleasant? When does it suit her to engage in movement, and how? When does she not want to? What kinds of associations and memories do movement and play bring up? All these experiences are not to be taken for granted in a girl who was subject to continued sexual abuse. The abuse 'accustomed' Shir to a reality in which she was prevented from paying attention to her needs and desires and even beyond this, erased them, erased herself.

In therapy, in contrast, she was given the option of choosing, to decide about herself, to be in control of the environment and reality. These significant experiences established, as time went on, a protected place and a safe relationship of trust, allowing her to share more from the depths of her soul. The movement release calmed her body and simultaneously, reduced the threat of a close relationship.

Living in trauma – Like a ship colliding with an iceberg

The word 'trauma' comes from the Greek word meaning 'wound', and in the particular case of sexual trauma, a psychic wound that plays out on the ground of the body. In adolescent girls, the traumatic wound typically emerges as a one-time assault, under which additional layers of abuse/ongoing injury are at times exposed. Every such assault can develop into post-traumatic stress disorder (PTSD) and in the case of ongoing abuse, into complex PTSD. In adolescent girls, sexual abuse occurs at a critical time in their life; as in every developmental stage, adolescence is also a crisis which creates systemic imbalance. Sexual abuse during this developmental period resembles a ship which has veered off course and collided with an iceberg. Systemic freezing occurs in the body and in life which, though it seems to continue, is stuck in the past. Levine (1997) notes that the core of the (traumatic) process is found in the immobility or freeze response; just as when the fight and flight responses are thwarted, the organism instinctively constricts and reacts by freezing. As the result of a traumatic event that threatened the physical integrity of the body and soul, body energy which could not be released in the movement of fighting and/or fleeing is trapped and this is the root of the formation of PTSD. In adolescent girls, the freeze response in inherent since it is implanted as part of the socialisation process with respect to their bodies (Young, 1980). For girls, the difficulty in responding in a motoric manner, that is, with a fight and/or flight movement, is intensified and as such, the probability increases that sexual assault will engender not only a traumatic experience, but also PTSD which will continue to impact their lives over time.

The impact is revealed in a variety of symptoms which may harm functioning – a re-experience of the event in an all-pervading way (flashbacks, painful memories, nightmares), avoidance of stimuli related to the trauma (avoiding thoughts, activities, people, places connected with the trauma), negative changes to cognition and mood (negative thoughts, exaggerated self-guilt and/or guilt of others, negative affect, sense of loneliness), and changes in the degree of arousal and reactivity (difficulty falling asleep and/or sleeping, restlessness, attention, and concentration difficulties, risky and/or destructive behaviour) (DSM5, APA, 2013).

The iceberg of a secret

A freeze defence response to sexual assault, in many cases, forms another iceberg – the iceberg of the secret. In the initial period following and/or during the assault (where abuse is ongoing), before the abuse is identified and exposed, a dissociative response which disconnects awareness from the here and now is active, full strength (Herman, 1992). The unconscious aim of dissociation is to prevent exposure of the secret and acknowledgement of the pain and suffering experienced (Cohen & Shacham, 2017). Sexual assault, unlike other types of assault (road accidents, terrorist attacks, war), occurs in seclusion, both literally and symbolically and as such, is kept secret, leaving the victim in a state of dreadful loneliness (Seligman & Solomon, 2004). The secret creates a two-fold distancing – of the victim from herself and of the victim from others. Thus, the secret produces a 'double life', split and dissociated.

On the one hand, the secret wants to be revealed, that is, there is a burning desire to expose, reveal, and share it with another person. On the other hand, in many cases, the profound and difficult experience is that there is no one to hear and contain the secret. The absence of a self-object recalls the unsafe attachment, which created a primal defensive state of encapsulation (Aharoni, 2005). The psychic iceberg of the secret thus continues to exist and to isolate the young girl from herself and her surroundings without the ability to thaw, change form, transform, and process. Beyond keeping the secret, the loneliness of teenage girls is also exacerbated owing to adolescents' experience of a generation gap vis-à-vis the adult world (Friedman, 2011). A natural need for privacy and separation, expressed at times in defiant and rebellious behaviour, and for sexually abused girls also takes on the sense of concealing and bottling up the secret. There is a greater likelihood of the secret being revealed among a group of the girl's peers which represents a place of sharing. In such cases, while the secret will be thawed and revealed it frequently remains without a proper response having been provided.

Anna, 12 years old, represents a situation in which the secret has no words but nonetheless, finds a way of being told through the body. Anna kept the secret of the abuse for several years. She kept the secret even from herself. She kept it bottled up inside. She did not let it out until it burst forth, uncontrollably. The first symptom to appear and attempt to 'tell' of the abuse was *encopresis*, faecal incontinence, this being the body's non-verbal somatic speech. Anna is an excellent dancer, in full control of her body, mainly in fight mode. At the time of the assault, she froze, was unable to move, unable to act, 'lost her voice' (Gilligan, 1982).

The process of revelation – The iceberg cracks

Discovering the secret is in itself a traumatic journey. The iceberg of dissociation detaches and protects against coherent, actual and threatening memory; however, it begins to thaw and break apart uncontrollably. The dam bursts and the memory transitions from freeze to flow to flood. In cases where the girl herself is detached, not conscious and does not remember the trauma she went through, the 'sky falls', what was will no longer be. The secret bursts through to memory and consciousness at once, through sensory flashbacks (smells, voices, feelings), in dreams and nightmares, in unexplainable memory fragments. This was how Michelle described the sudden memories of sexual abuse she went through.

Michelle, 13 years old, discovered her abuse during a 'sex education' lesson in school. In a single moment, an image of him touching her burst into her awareness. She did not believe it: 'This can't be', she said, 'how it is that I didn't remember this for so many years'?! 'Maybe I'm imagining'?! There is no continuity. Memory fragments floated up. Michelle preferred to forget but her body spoke. Each time the assault was remembered, her mouth became dry, her eyes froze, her hands began to move restlessly, bunching up the pouffe in the treatment room. I explain about the body's response and how much it is tied to what she underwent and tells of the assault, and she is surprised, not always ready to accept that her body is a full partner. When the environment begins to recognise, a response of belief, validation, and reinforcement which respects the pace of the victim and is sensitive to her needs, can lead to a process of healing. In contrast, a response which minimises the abuse, casts doubt, is angry, accusatory, denying and ignoring leads to a long and painful journey with a harsher prognosis for recovery. At times, the environment's response to the discovery of the secret is the most difficult experience which may eventually become a trauma itself (Szwarcberg & Somer, 2004).

The manner of the mother's response to discovery of the secret of the abuse is critical for the girl. In adolescence, the mother's role in the girl's life intensifies and the two become entangled (Friedman, 2011), and are simultaneously involved in dual relations of connection and disconnection, closeness and distancing. With sexual assault, the girl's closeness with her mother is essential because, often, it is linked to a predisposition to assault. That is to say, it is an important component in the communication-dynamic conditions in which the girl is growing up and is a significant part of the context in which the assault took place. Along with the complexity, during the course of therapy, mother-daughter relations can become a central resource in the healing process. A mother whose daughter was a victim of sexual assault is necessarily also harmed in at least two ways: one, there is a good chance that she too was sexually assaulted; the second is inherent in the guilt she carries in relation to the parental failure to protect her daughter. It has been found that among mothers who were victims of incest, there is eight-fold greater risk of their daughter or son being a victim of abuse during their lifetime (Gur, 2014). That is, at times, the daughter's abuse constitutes part of an unconscious dynamic of intergenerational transfer. Another recently revealed finding showed a kind of reverse intergenerational process according to which mothers of girls who were sexually assaulted, and who supported their daughters during the course of discovery and treatment of the assault, were discovered to suffer from post-traumatic symptoms familiar from the world of sexual abuse despite them not having been abused themselves (Mordish Volk, 2021).

It is important to encourage, strengthen, cultivate, and deepen the relationship with the mother according to the girl's need, desire, and pace. Along with this, at times, the experience of the mother's betrayal of the daughter, in that she did not prevent the abuse and protect her, is so profound to the point where it is hard to repair the break and re-establish relations of trust between them (Gur, 2014). In a crisis situation such as when sexual abuse is discovered, relations with the mother can bestow upon the daughter security, protection, trust, assistance, and reliance, strengthening the girl on deep levels in her attachment relationship and helping her restore her self, her strengths. In this sense, the mother can represent a beneficent 'self-object' (Kohut, 1984) in the discovery and healing journey. The following vignette from Shir's therapy presents complex mother-daughter relations, as a process parallel to the deep connection between Shir and her dog.

Shir brings her dog Sheila to one of the sessions. In their relations, Shir is the mother and Sheila is the daughter. Shir does not feel well during the session. Her eyes are shiny; I warm her up with tea and a blanket. She is after a busy period of much schoolwork and lies down on the pouffe and relaxes. Suddenly, Sheila pees. I normalise this and reframe her behaviour as discharging tension as a result of excitement and anxiety about being in a new place. Shir, on the other hand, not only scolds her, but also explains and interprets her: 'She was also subject to trauma, her tail is broken and that's why we don't know when she's happy. It bothers my mother because she looks sad all the time'.

I understand that here there is an enactment of relations tied to the sexual trauma and perhaps also with Shir's primal attachment to her mother. Suddenly, Shir takes Sheila, turns her upside down, and picks her up from her legs. Sheila freezes and her eyes are panicked, but Shir ignores this. She forces her to play games she doesn't like; she says she is not smart enough and that she is a dog with attention disorders, just like her. At one of the sessions, Shir fears that Sheila is pregnant and talks crudely about her: 'she's in heat, she wants it'. On the other hand, she cannot be without her for a moment and is very devoted to her. Sheila relieves her loneliness and Shir makes sure she eats, drinks, that her bowl is clean. Shir sits on the soft pouffe, submerges herself in it, and moulds it. She and Sheila snuggle up with one another, and this allows Shir to relax. The energy is released and she spontaneously takes deep breaths. In parallel, over the long course of therapy, Shir and her mother manage to communicate in words and fight less. Shir: 'At least I stayed sane. Even Mum tells me that despite the difficult things I went through I'm stronger than it seems'.

Shame and guilt over the freeze

The stage of identifying the assault should provide relief, thawing, a return to going on being (Winnicott, 1960). However, alongside the fact that the abuse generally ceases once it is uncovered, calm is not yet attained. The moment of discovery is a traumatic and freezing stage which raises difficult and constricting emotions of shame and guilt. These emotions appear in the body and movement – introversion, contraction, reduction of the kinespheric space, and reduction of movement in the space. That is, not using the full potential of the body and movement (Young, 1980).

The guilt relates to the act itself, to forbidden sexuality according to social codes and frequently, according to the law as well, and to the permission and/or agreement that the girl 'seemingly' gave to the abuser, since she could not do anything to prevent her abuse. The shame is related to the self – to 'who I am'. This is one of the profound, tenacious, and soul-killing damages of sexual trauma and it includes shame concerning 'who I am', the sense of defectiveness, revulsion from the body and from the self (Naveh, 2020).

For girls, shame is also linked to gender belonging, to the fact that the assault occurred to their body as girls, women-to-be, and also to the fact that this is a violation of a sexual nature. Personal and societal preoccupation with the body and sexuality, particularly among teenage girls, is characterised by socialisation processes of double and occasionally contradictory messages which sow deep confusion from a values and identity perspective (Weinberg & Tamir, 2017). The subject of sexuality among teenage girls is, on the one hand, socially taboo, a topic which, seemingly, is forbidden to discuss since it arouses strong feelings of shame, embarrassment, and guilt. On the other hand, it is a 'sexy' and popular topic so much so that it is impossible not to relate to it. The media and the media industry create the awareness among the population of girls that they are judged, first and foremost, by their external appearance. Consumer goods aim to externalise their feminine sexuality so that on the outside, they look 'like grown women', and perpetuate the 'little women' oxymoron. In parallel, the notion that it is not acceptable for a girl to initiate, desire, and enjoy sexuality is also extant in the collective mind, despite that at times, girls' liberated preoccupation with their body and sexuality actually attests to their awareness of freedom of choice and not necessarily to a preoccupation resulting from patriarchal oppression (Duitz & van Zoonen, 2006).

Davidson and Ribak (2017) examined the question of whether girls have a choice about whether to be a 'slut'. That is to say, does a girl have the right and freedom to choose the way she behaves and presents herself sexually? The answer to this question is deceptive especially in light of two competing images in social discourse with reference to girls. One focuses on the image of 'girl power', which is tied to free choice and to the elevation of the body and the mind, while the other is linked to the concept of 'at-risk girls', that is, a conception of girls as a disadvantaged sector of society which must be protected and safeguarded through oppressive socialisation that dictates feelings of shame and guilt with respect to the body and sexuality (Aapola, Gonick, & Harris, 2005).

The discourse regarding girls who were sexually violated most often reinforces the social position of victimisation and threat, that is, the conception of girls as naïve, vulnerable, endangered, and 'voiceless' (Brown & Gilligan, 1992), and relates to them less in the vein of 'girl power', as having the power to resist and to create social change. The loss of childhood experienced by girls who were sexually assaulted is two-fold. One is experienced due to the bodily changes that occur during adolescence which are not controllable and can frequently arouse feelings of powerlessness, disgust, and fear. The second is experienced as a result of the assault, in which the girl becomes an object, a tool in the hands of another person, for his needs alone (Seligman, 2004).

Sexual assault of girls does not correspond to their emotional developmental stage. It does not satisfy their need for tenderness and love but forces inappropriate desire upon them (Ferenczi, 1933/1949). Different girls will react differently but there are two core common reactions: one will be expressed in an automatic linkage between touch and sexuality and an experience of violation. Every touch will set her off, and every attempt at closeness will lead to vigilance and over-arousal. Every touch to the body, even for purposes of pleasure and enjoyment, will be experienced as humiliating and painful. The second reaction is seemingly the opposite, a protective response of reaction formation that will be expressed in the appearance of disconnection from bodily experience and 'seductive behaviour'. That is, using the body in order to create a connection, to draw attention, due to a self-perception of 'I'm only good with my body'. In the final analysis, both types of reaction arouse awful shame and with both, the body is experienced as an object and not as an integral part on the continuum of the self.

The vignette below relates to the re-victimisation phenomenon among sexually abused girls. Paradoxically, the fact of a first assault increases the probability that the girl will be assaulted again. Oftentimes, girls who were sexually assaulted will, out of their distress, again attach themselves to people who take advantage of them and assault them. It is the only relationship pattern they know, and they 'prefer' to be in an abusive relationship than to remain lonely. This is the re-victimisation mechanism, which repeatedly recreates the assault (Seligman, 2004), a non-adaptive behaviour pattern in which the lonely girl seeks tenderness, but encounters destructive desire.

During the course of therapy, Shir is again assaulted. She appears to 'offer' her body, appears to 'ask' to be harmed. Her boyfriend didn't answer his phone and Mum didn't answer either. Shir was in distress and she turned to the first person who offered her physical closeness. With intense loneliness and the inability to regulate it, a 'confusion of the tongues' sets in – the native language of tenderness and the language of desire from the adult world (Ferenczi, 1933/1949). As a result of this new assault, Shir wanted to die. She ran amok all through her school, wanting to 'turn back the clock', but she could not. Her boyfriend already knew. She felt that she had ruined her life. When she comes to me she blames herself: 'I have a serious problem here in my head (she hits her head). With how I think. I get to places I don't want to be in and I don't even know what I was doing there'. She speaks in a torrent, courageously and consciously. Shir makes the connection between the fresh assault and the ongoing abuse of her childhood and generates meaning: 'He didn't listen and I stopped speaking. I froze. A sense that you're trying to feel your legs but you can't. I try to move my arms but I can't. I try to make my mouth speak but I can't. And what happened this time is exactly the same thing. I didn't behave according to how I felt, I didn't understand what was happening to me. How did I go there'?

She begins to use writing as a platform for thawing. Writing as a means to renew the sequence of memories and the natural flow of the self: 'It was hard to write', she says. 'I actually had a panic attack when I began. My body tried to prevent me from remembering. I felt fear, shivers'. I reframe this in a somewhat different context and say: 'But it was actually the body – those shivers – that helped you remember what happened then, when you were eight'. Shir answers: 'I stopped listening to myself, because no one listened to me then … I didn't understand what he wanted from me. I couldn't do anything'. Shir agrees to work with her body and to try and learn from it about the inner story of her psyche. She seats herself on the easy chair, does not lean back but sits with her weight forward and talks about herself: 'It's like, so that I can escape quickly'. While she talks I understand how hard it is for her, but I also recognise that now she protects herself more, she is alert to fear, prepares to flee. 'What do you pay attention to'? I ask. 'A strange sense of detachment. Heaviness in my lower abdomen. My head is empty of thoughts. It's weird … and there's no emotion …', she answers.

Though Shir feels detached, she describes bodily sensations which attest to the connection she has developed to the felt sense, to becoming aware to the physical sensations of the body and the situation (Levine, 1997). She manages to dwell and not immediately act, something that never happened before. Several moments later, she yawns, breathes deeply, stretches. I explain to her that this is a spontaneous discharge of energy, that her body is intelligent and her nervous system regulates itself. Locked energy which froze gradually becomes released (Levine, 1997). I am inclined to view Shir's repeated assault as part of a maladaptive attempt to 'treat' the awful loneliness she was feeling.

In addition to harmful connections, adolescent girls who were sexually abused often try out a variety of self-harming, suicidal and non-suicidal behaviours – outbursts of rage, suicidality, injury, eating disorders (as slow and ongoing suicide), alcohol and drug use, 'seduction' using the body and sexuality for self-regulation and calming purposes, and nowadays, self-harm broadcast via social media – with the aim of getting as many 'likes' as possible even at the expense of bodily and mental exposure. Any behaviour that has the power to dull the unbearable psychic pain and to detach from it – cutting, drug use, obsessive preoccupation with eating, sex, angry outbursts – all are seemingly legitimate from their perspective (Davies & Frawley, 1994).

One of the goals of therapy is, together with the teenage girl, to try and understand these behaviours, both the harmful and ineffective aspects and their source. Therapy helps raise awareness to the distress and the desire to take action in any possible way – by fight or flight, the main thing being not to freeze or to faint (play dead) (Levine, 1997), as automatically happened to them during the traumatic event.

Girls relate that after the assault they sometimes felt they were 'going mad', that there was something abnormal about them. Their emotional lability which, in any case is exaggerated among adolescents, is exacerbated among girls who have been abused. The core of therapy in this aspect is normalising the feeling of 'madness' by providing a logical explanation for extreme reactions that occur in the attempt to survive, as well as restoring a normal reaction to an abnormal situation such as they experienced in the assault. This, along with engaging in bodily experiences and beneficial movement, can facilitate regulation and calm and guide feelings of compassion towards themselves and at times, reduce harmful behaviours. The case of Ella demonstrates the vulnerable situation of a girl who attempted a maladaptive self-treatment of self-harm.

Ella, 15 years old, came to therapy due to stomach aches and vomiting which attacked her at social gatherings. At the second session, she already reveals a secret to me – for some time she has been cutting herself with the removable blade of a pencil sharpener. After a number of sessions, another secret is revealed – of a sexual assault she experienced two years earlier perpetrated by a boy her age who 'wanted to hook up with me'. When she did not comply, he disseminated embarrassing photos of her via WhatsApp. I work with her using subtle interventions associated with the 'somatic experience' approach and ask her about her sense of her body at this moment: 'The soles of my feet are becoming numb. My jaw is stuck. Words aren't coming out. I think them in my head but the words don't come out of my mouth … in me, the entire area connected to breathing and vomiting are active (Ella suffers from bronchial asthma and skin asthma), chest and throat … when I imagine slapping my ex-boyfriend, it does me good'.

Ella is warming up and recalls a childhood memory:

> When I was nine, I was against boys on principle. There was a boy who really annoyed me and I let him have it. I scratched him, don't remember why. I was afraid to tell my parents and I kept it secret. They only found out when I was suspended from school.

Ella once again enters a freeze situation and says: 'Today, when I get angry – I keep quiet'. I point out the connection to the cutting and 'make sense' of her remarks:

> Silence is like a cut, turning the anger inward, that's where the anger drains in to. Here, we're trying to let the anger out. You're not at fault for what happened.

Movement completion technique

The rage accumulated in the body from the freeze and trapped in the body (Levine, 1997) during the traumatic event can be released by means of a 'movement completion' technique. The movement which froze during the threatening incident is realised in therapy – in reality and/or in imagination. In another case description demonstrating this, Laurie and her sister were assaulted by a close neighbour-friend of the family. The moment Laurie discovered that her younger sister was also assaulted, she decided to lodge a complaint with the police. Mainly, she wanted to protect her younger sister, less perceiving herself as abused: 'My sister was much more harmed than I', she said. Laurie is her home's security guard, the fighter.

> I'm Mum's rock ... I always know what to do in emergency situations. When my sister attempted suicide, I acted immediately, I called for help. Mum screamed and cried, she didn't know what to do, and I functioned in her place ... it was only during the assault that I froze ... that's what makes me the angriest, that he's walking around free and not paying the price. I want to take revenge on him and on the other hand, I can't, I'm afraid that I may make a mistake or do something stupid and afterwards, I'll pay the price.

Laurie shares a dream she dreamt: 'I was trapped in some car. I was kidnapped and tied to the seat. I felt trapped, that I was losing control. The men there were violent'.

We work with the body and pay attention to the feeling. It appears that much rage remains in the body with reference to the powerlessness to act, about the secret that was kept, about the offender who is freely walking around, about not preventing her sister's abuse: 'I want to pay him back! So that he feels what it's like'. Her legs are charged with the energy of anger, of frustration, and I suggest that she, for a moment, contract her whole body and then release. She does so and feels relief. Suddenly she breathes. Laurie is in fight mode, powerfully kicks the inflatable bobo doll, but all is done in silence. She has no voice.

In Laurie's case, the difficulty in making her voice heard did not appear initially during the assault when she froze but rather, is part of the familial gender dynamic. 'When I was little, in the neighbourhood I'd be called names because I always hung around with boys. I always perceived myself as similar to boys because I was physically strong. Until today, I have this kind of build. Today, I already want to get dressed up, but I'm anxious that it won't look good on me. In my eyes, I don't look sexy or attractive ...'.

Laurie is an unusually beautiful teenager. Her eyes are light, her hair long and flowing, a solid body build, her legs are muscular and her shoulders are somewhat broad, a 'fighter'. Together with her, I wonder why even today, as a teenager and not a child, her self-image is of someone who resembles a boy. Another question comes up, 'why can't a woman be both strong and beautiful'?! Laurie explains that her older brother is the 'prince' at home, an only son who receives preferential treatment from his parents. He takes the role of the 'protector' and is over-protective of her, does not allow any male friend to get close to her and limits her in the choice of boys with whom she can meet. He invades her boundaries, dominates, meddles in the type of clothing she wears, and does not allow her to grow up and experience a romantic relationship. In spite of his good intentions, her brother's protection is, at times, experienced more as violation than safeguarding and protective. Laurie describes: 'With boys, let's say someone positions his arm as if to give me a hug, right away, I become tense and push his arm away. It reminds me of the offender and also I think about whether my brother would allow it. Boys often think that they're allowed to do anything'. Presented with this content, I think of the atmosphere of her home. The power is in the hands of the men, and the women's voices are not heard, silenced. In this sense, Laurie's voice and that of her sister were twice not heard – during the assault and at home.

Transference relations in therapy with abused adolescent girls

Frequently, in work with sexually abused victims, and particularly with teenage girls, the dynamic in the abuse relations is re-enacted in therapy in transference relations between the therapist and the girl. According to Davies and Frawley (1994), unconscious enactment in the 'here and now' is another attempt to cope with the assault. Through projective identification processes in which actual, raw physical feelings of weakness, freezing, helplessness, fear, use of force, use of authority, diminishing of the other, erasing and disregarding the other's needs are unconsciously projected onto the therapist, it becomes possible to understand the girl's subjective experience of abuse. The therapist takes on the 'thing in itself' (Bion, 1970), that is, actual re-enactment of parts of interaction from the core of the abusive relations. This initially reduces the therapeutic space but later, through mentalisation and the therapist's attribution of meaning to the enactment of the abusive relations, it will expand and receive deeper meaning.

The field of abuse is toxic and in order to provide treatment, there is no other way than experiencing it on our own person. Here, the teenage girl's need comes into play – to experience the therapist as a 'real person', as a woman with attitudes and opinions, also able to act and exist outside the therapy bubble. In this sense, treating abused teenage girls demands, to a great extent, systemic work (welfare and education entities, parents) and being available outside of therapy. It is important for the girls to know and sense that the therapist is 'there for them', obviously within the holding, containing, and personal boundaries of each therapist. The following case will demonstrate an enactment of abusive relations in therapy.

Shir's patchwork quilt

I notice that I have much tension and arousal prior to sessions with Shir. I try to contain the difficult feelings flung into me. This time Shir arrives ticked off. She is restless, moving quickly, angry at me. She creates all sorts of things quickly and then throws them away, cleans, punctures, cuts, pours, peels, uses large amounts of art materials ... she is fuming. The slime doesn't come out like it's supposed to. She says she is under great pressure at school, and she fears being trapped here forever. I understand that in the 'here and now', the therapy and I, from her perspective, are re-enacting the control, coercion, and inattentiveness to her desires and needs, just as in the assault. I am the abuser and she is the abused and vice versa. I try to speak and she responds in shouts: 'Oh come on, enough Orna, I already told you that I don't want to talk about it'!!! I am silenced. Afraid, helpless, I have no words, don't know what to do, and what will thaw the iceberg between us.

I suddenly feel profound sadness, I imagine Shir as a child. How alone she was, how alone she is today, even at this moment. I say: 'No one is forced to come here. It's under your control'. Shir listens to me, softens, and we come closer with our eyes. Several sessions later she asks to create a pillow in the shape of a donut for her room at home. I understand this to be something soft that she wants to take from the room, from the relationship. She saw how to make the pillow on YouTube and I agree to her request. I buy her suitable fabric and bring sewing tools for her despite not really knowing how to do this and not being particularly talented, but we complement one another. Shir is good at cutting and I at sewing. We sit close to each other. An association of a mother and daughter comes up, playing together, creating a patchwork quilt. Shir does not sew because she is afraid of needles. At her initiative, in a shaky voice, she shares her fear of separation from her mother who is about to undergo surgery. Shir does not want to end the session and I say: 'If it were possible, we would stay here together all day long'.

In summary, DMT with adolescent girls who were sexually abused is a powerful experience for all involved – the girl, her family, and the therapist. It is an agitating experience comprising a triangular therapeutic ground: one side is the developmental period of adolescence. The second side is the harsh and extreme impact which sexual abuse generally has on all areas of life. The third side is linked to preoccupation with the body and movement. These three dimensions tend to intensify and amplify almost every layer in therapy, for better and for worse. They create a very high level of sensitivity, which brings up intense and extreme emotions within the relationship for both the therapist and the patient. At the same time, there are 'magical moments' of joint dancing as a basis for development of trust and emotional intimacy. Progress in this type of therapy is not linear, but shifts in every which way and in diverse ways, precarious, empowering, moving, and full of love.

The use of somatic and movement work, as described in the case descriptions, can occasionally arouse opposition among girls who have been abused. The reluctance generally derives from a fear of being in close contact with the same body that was assaulted, violated, that is impossible to safeguard, from which they constantly tried to disconnect. Yet, the opposite is true. It is actually the experience of listening to the body and to sensations, familiarity with the body, a movement warmup of the body and joints, relaxation techniques, listening to the breath, the ability to linger in non-movement, listening to freeze, completing movement, giving space and reinforcement to explosive strength, contraction and relaxation, grounding, release, free movement in the room, games involving movement – which enable these girls to reclaim their bodies and souls (Alvarez, 1992). These experiences can open a window of opportunities to thaw the body and psyche from the traumatic freeze towards the free flow of life.

Acknowledgements

My gratitude to the girls as it has been a privilege to accompany along the way, thanks to whom I learned and am still learning about love in therapy. Thank you to my dear friends and colleagues at the 'Maor' Centre. Our partnership has created for me a stable environment of comradeship, benevolence, and the friendship of sisterhood. A deeply heartfelt thank you to Avramit Brodsky, my special supervisor, from whom I learn each time anew how to be a better person and therapist. And an immense thank you to Maor director, Dr. Efrat Naveh, who has been raising me and empowering me for many years.

References

Aapola, S., Gonick, M., & Harris, A. (2005). *Young femininity: Girlhood, power and social change* (1st ed.). London: Palgrave Macmillan.

Aharoni, H. (2005). A closely guarded secret: From an attentive ear to a containing mind. *Sichot, 19*(2), 159–167 (Hebrew).

Alvarez, A. (1992). *Live company: Psychoanalytic psychotherapy with autistic, borderline, deprived and abused children.* New York, NY: Brunner Routledge.

American Psychiatric Association. (2013). *Diagnostic and statistical manual of mental disorders* (5th ed.). Washington, DC: APA.

Bion, W. R. (1970). *Attention and interpretation.* London: Tavistock Publications Ltd.

Brown, L., & Gilligan, C. (1992). *Meeting at the crossroads: Women's psychology and girls' development*. Cambridge, MA: Harvard University Press.

Cohen, L. & Shacham, M. (2017). The phenomenon of physical detachment in movement therapy with victims of incest. Between the words, 13, 20–25. (Hebrew).

Davidson, S., & Ribak, R. (2017). 'Let everyone see my body': Online photo sharing and rating among adolescent girls. In E. Lachover, E. Peled, & M. Komem (Eds.), *Girls and their bodies. Voice, presence, absence* (pp. 43–65). Jerusalem: Magnes, The Hebrew University of Jerusalem (Hebrew).

Davies, J. M., & Frawley, M. G. (1994). *Treating the adult survivor of childhood sexual abuse*. New York, NY: Basic Books.

Dell, C. (1970). *A primer for movement description. Using effort/shape and supplementary concepts*. New York: Dance Notation Bureau.

Duitz, L., & van Zoonen, L. (2006). Head scarves and porno chic: Disciplining girls' bodies in the European multicultural society. *European Journal of Women's Studies*, 13(2), 103–117.

Elior, R. (2010). 'Present but absent', 'Still life', and 'A pretty maiden who has no eyes': On the presence and absence of women in the Hebrew language, in the Jewish religion, and Israeli life. *Studies in Spirituality*, 20, 381–455.

Ferenczi, S. (1949). Confusion of the tongues between the adults and the child – (The language of tenderness and of passion) (Michael Balint, Trans.). *International Journal of Psycho-Analysis*, 30, 225–230 (Original work published 1933).

Friedman, A. (2011). *Connected – Mothers and daughters*. Tel Aviv: Modan (Hebrew)

Gilligan, C. (1982). *In a different voice: Psychological theory and women's development*. Cambridge, MA: Harvard University Press.

Gur, A. (2014). *Mothers and children at the edge of the risk continuum*. Lecture delivered February 22, 2007, published on https://wtc-anatgur.co.il (Hebrew).

Herman, J. L. (1992). *Trauma and recovery: The aftermath of violence – From domestic abuse to political terror*. New York, NY: Basic Books.

Kohut, H. (1984). *How does analysis cure?* Edited by Arnold Goldberg with the collaboration of Paul E. Stepansky. Chicago, IL: University of Chicago Press.

Laban, R., & Lawrence, F. C. (1947). *Effort*. London: Duckworth.

Levine, P. A. (1997). *Waking the tiger: Healing trauma: The innate capacity to transform overwhelming experiences*. Berkeley, CA: North Atlantic Books.

Mordish Volk, N. (2021). *The helping connection: how mothers of daughters who were sexually abused experience the relationship to their daughter's therapist* [PhD thesis], Be'er Sheva, Ben-Gurion University (Hebrew).

Naveh, A. (2020). *The shock with the discovery of sexual abuse inside and outside the family*. From a lecture for protected teams at the Yoav Regional Council, December 29, 2020 (Hebrew).

Porges, S. W. (2011). *The polyvagal theory: Neuropsychological foundations of emotions, attachment, communication and self-regulation*. New York: Norton.

Seligman, Z. (2004). Witnessing in the treatment of trauma and incest: Re-embodiment and re-analysis of the trauma in light of transference and countertransference. In Z. Seligman & Z. Solomon (Eds.), *Critical and clinical perspectives on incest* (pp. 240–256). Tel Aviv: Hakibbutz Hameuchad/Adler Center – Tel Aviv University (Hebrew).

Seligman, Z., & Solomon, Z. (2004). *Critical and clinical perspectives in incest*. Tel Aviv: Hakibbutz Hameuchad/Adler Center – Tel Aviv University (Hebrew).

Shuper Engelhard, E. (2014). Dance/movement therapy during adolescence: Learning about adolescence through the experiential movement of dance/movement therapy students. *Arts in Psychotherapy*, *41*, 498–503.

Szwarcberg, S., & Somer, E. (2004). Disclosure of the secret: Facilitating and inhibiting variables in the disclosure of child sexual abuse. In Z. Seligman & Z. Solomon (Eds.), *Critical and clinical perspectives in incest* (pp. 1–577). Tel Aviv: Hakibbutz Hameuchad/Adler Center – Tel Aviv University (Hebrew).

Weinberg, D., & Tamir, T. (2017). Girls in essence': Insights from work with girls and with staff on body, health and sexuality. In E. Lachover, E. Peled, & M. Komem (Eds.), *Girls and their bodies. voice, presence, absence* (pp. 43–65). Jerusalem: Magnes, The Hebrew University of Jerusalem (Hebrew).

Winnicott, D. W. (1960). The theory of the parent-infant relationship. *International Journal of Psychoanalysis*, *41*, 585–595.

Young, I. (1980). Throwing like a girl: A phenomenology of feminine body comportment, motility and spatiality. *Human Studies*, *3*, 137–156.

Ziv, E. (2012). Insidious trauma. *Mafteach – Ktav-et Lexicali LeMachshava Politit*, *5*, 55–74 (Hebrew).

Chapter 4

A Renewed Observation of the Treatment of Sexual Abuse in a Therapeutic Setting for Eating Disorders

Maayan Dor Haim

Introduction

This chapter discusses central issues in the treatment of adolescent girls who suffer from both eating disorders and sexual assault. In the writing of this chapter, 25 case descriptions were re-examined of adolescent girls who suffered from a combination of sexual abuse and an eating disorder. The chapter is interspersed with case descriptions and discusses the contribution of Bioenergetic Analysis and Dance Movement Therapy (DMT) and their significance given in parallel to verbal psychotherapy.

In my work as a dance-movement therapist in a therapeutic setting dedicated to eating disorders, some of the adolescent girls I encountered had experienced sexual abuse. I looked back from a new perspective at the therapies with girls who suffered from eating disorders and had experienced sexual abuse, to attempt to re-examine and conceptualise insights in this context. In retrospection of over 25 years of treatment of adolescents with eating disorders, I chose to examine 25 case studies written in the last 15 years. I organised these cases in a table, adding and eliminating columns according to what I found. Collecting the cases and observing them through a lens focused on sexual abuse brought to light significant issues and themes, which I will present, addressing the verbal and non-verbal expression that occurs in DMT conducted concurrently with psychotherapy.

Much has been written about sexual abuse, eating disorders, and DMT. In my in-depth review of the cases I had treated, in qualitative as well as quantitative terms, the centrality of the concepts from the mind-movement paradigm (Shahar-Levy, 2005) and bioenergetic analysis (Lowen, 1976) to an understanding of the therapeutic process, became progressively evident. In therapies where meaningful change seemed to have occurred through working with the body, significant transition was apparent: from the movement of the parental envelope paradigm to the movement of the vertical face-to-face paradigm, and from grounding into oneself (on the vertical plane) to relational grounding (on the horizontal plane).

DOI: 10.4324/9781003309048-7

Shahar-Levy (2005) viewed the parental envelope space and the vertical face-to-face space as a set of universal interpersonal relationships reflected in different forms on the bodily, relational, and communications plane of reality. In the parental envelope setting (referred to as P0), the self is held within the parental envelope, protected and enclosed by it in early life, through touch, movement, and voice. The parental envelope has the functions of carrying, nourishing, and protecting; it serves as a sort of physical and emotional sequel to the envelope of the womb. The infant's body needs its parents' protection to contend with the force of gravity, and is utterly dependent on them. In this relational setting, there is no differentiation, from the infant's perspective, between the enclosed body of the self and the enclosing body of the other.

The parental envelope setting is imprinted in the body memory of the infant and encoded as a pattern internalised within its body image. In the vertical face-to-face setting (referred to as P1), the self exists and faces others independently and autonomously. Concurrently with the motor development process and the separation-individuation process, in parallel to its psychological birth, the infant separates from the parental envelope setting and transitions to a vertical face-to-face setting. The infant holds itself upright, using its muscles and skeleton, in the face of gravity, and confronts the other with forceful energy. This setting is the foundation for the experience of resilience of the self, autonomy, and separateness.

Throughout life, these two sets of movement paradigms are in dialogue – a discourse between the parental envelope and the vertical face-to-face relational languages. In normal development, transitions between these emotional movement languages are interwoven to create enhanced flexibility and the ability to take pleasure in different forms of attachment. In pathological development, the language of one movement space may dominate, leading to conflicts or creating barriers blocking the body and movement from the internal emotional experience. The case studies presented below illuminate the extent to which the possibility for a space allowing transition from the dominance of either language – parental envelope or vertical face-to-face – to an integration of both languages is crucial to development in therapy.

Lowen (1976) saw grounding as a developmental process of self-awareness, self-expression, and self-possession. Lowen defines vitality as an experience of expansion of the organism and the flow of energy from the core to the periphery. This is the movement of the true self, where continuity of being is maintained. Being grounded in reality, for Lowen, is equivalent to Winnicott's concept of the true self. The capacity to experience the self (self-awareness), the ability to express emotions (self-expression), and the ability to contain oneself (self-possession) reflects Lowen's energetic concepts of grounding – the possibility of expansion, pleasure, and movement towards the other, as well as delay, restraint, and modulation. When the self retreats from physical or mental pain, it signals danger, and a disruption in the continuity of being emerges. In this situation, the infant or toddler is forced to hold themselves, leading to the development of a false self. Despite the loss of vitality of the true self, self-holding protects it (from fear of falling, or fear of breakdown), in the absence of a holding environment. The ability to exist in reality is only possible if the self is relatively free of excessive defensiveness. A defensive organisation is designed to reduce pain and anxiety, and to compensate for what is lacking. It is an experience of an absence of grounding, associated with a tendency to dissociation, fantasy, and loss of contact with reality of the grounded self.

Grounding is a deep element of energetic, somatic, emotional, and spiritual organisation of the self. On the vertical plane, grounding into oneself (self-awareness, self-expression, and self-possession) also encompasses the world beyond the human individual: the sky and the earth; and on the horizontal plane, relational grounding, meaning grounding to the other. The foetus takes root in the mother's body in pregnancy. The interchange between the horizontal and vertical planes, as they develop in tandem, continues to nurture both throughout life.

A meaningful transition in therapies conducted through the body relates to the movement from secure grounding into oneself, on the vertical axis, to secure relational grounding, on the horizontal axis. Fortifying and building the ability to recognise trauma and bear the awareness of it in the mind and body, to be anchored in the true self, creates the possibility for future self-expression – in other words, for unloading (verbally and bodily) in the presence of another. The process of anchoring trauma in the self – the ability to contain, experience, and express – with another, and to experience the connection with the other as a safe place, is crucial to development in therapy.

Different modes of being helped through dance movement therapy

In the therapies I will describe, the girls were treated with DMT and psychotherapy concurrently. This is a unique setting that engages the ability to form a connection and accept help in two different therapies. The different and unique dynamics and uses of DMT are highlighted against this background. Of the 25 cases, for some patients the combination of psychotherapy and DMT was complementary, enhancing the therapeutic effect and enriching the treatment with other qualities and different perspectives. For others, a split formed between the psychotherapy and the DMT.

Of the cases where a split between the therapies emerged, in four cases the patient cooperated in psychotherapy, while in one case the patient was primarily cooperative in DMT. The extreme form of this split occurred when paralysis and a lack of movement appeared in DMT, to the point of utter silence of the body (two cases). In two other cases, dominance of the emotional movement language of the parental envelope setting (P0) was observed in the DMT, or in Lowen's terms, grounding into oneself. In one case, the vertical face-to-face language (P1) was dominant – in Lowen's terms, defensive relational grounding (aggressive, with compulsive exercise). In cases where transition was possible between the paradigms of the parental envelope setting and the vertical face-to-face setting, and grounding into the self was possible in the presence of the other – in other words, the ability to contain, experience, and express was present – development in therapy through the body became possible (13 of the cases). In one case, where coop- eration emerged in P1 language, without the creation of trust in the relation- ship, the transition to P0 language was not secure and grounded. Through the case descriptions that follow, I will illustrate these qualities, as well as expressions of different modes of the ability to accept help in DMT. All iden- tifying information has been thoroughly altered to protect patient privacy. The cases will illuminate the way DMT supports the healing process, even when resistance to movement arises on the surface level.

Emotional flooding in psychotherapy and paralysis in dance movement therapy

In the first case study, I demonstrate a situation of cooperation in psycho- therapy, with qualities of emotional flooding, and an experience of paral- ysis in DMT – avoidance and an absence of movement: the silence of the body. Anna, a 16-year-old girl, suffered from post-traumatic stress disorder and from an eating disorder. When therapy began, she was in a severe depressive state. She did not speak, until the day she revealed prolonged sexual trauma. She suffered from flashbacks and suicidal ideation, and manifested extreme behaviours in relation to her body image, including sleeping clothed and avoidance of bathing.

Anna said she was not interested in DMT; the last thing she wanted, she stated, was to connect to her body. She had danced as a child, but did not remember the specifics. In fact, she could not remember childhood at all. At some point, things changed, she whispered. She appeared to be in distress; she said that it was hard for her to be with a stranger with the door to the room closed. Anna evoked a need to protect and soothe, and to prom- ise that we would move slowly and gradually. She refused to remove her shoes, sitting cross-legged on the floor until her immobile legs were numb. Her legs were exposed, wounded, and she was clearly uncomfortable. She accepted a soft ball from me and squeezed it. Her movements were small, close to the body, at the ends of her body (small range, motionless – P0). This was the only possibility for movement in the room. If the ball escaped her and rolled away, she would not reach out or stretch to bring it back.

She told me what she found calming: talking in psychotherapy, her sister, sudoku, and music. In DMT, we listened together to the music she chose. Anna struggled to trust me or lean on me, but she used me when she felt pressured, to obtain special treatment. Confronted with her suffering and the need to tread gently, it was difficult to set boundaries for her and disappoint her. At every session she came into the room with her shoes on and sat in the exact same spot; it was as though that was the extent of the space she had allotted herself. She spoke in whispers, or in gestures I struggled to interpret. She was tense, startled by every sound. Anna's minute movements shifted from squeezing to jabbing with her fingers (more powerful and direct – budding P1). The range of the possible for her being was extremely restricted. Each time we seemed to have found a potential mode of shared movement, or things were slightly more comfortable, she could not allow continuity and evolution in the following sessions (disjointedness – P0). She came to the sessions submissively. It was important to her to make her refusal known and have it accepted, but there was a price: her defensive and avoidant stance negated the possibility of progress.

In one session, she looked at the wounds on her legs, sliding her finger around them, careful not to injure herself or possibly considering hurting herself, as though referencing the elephant in the room. When I walked outdoors with her, she was more relaxed. She shared her wish to be a researcher, affording me a momentary glance at her strengths.

Having endured sexual trauma, Anna found the thought of being in therapy that addressed the body threatening in its own right, in the sense that any kind of connection with her body might recreate the trauma, which could not be digested. In a state of shock, she stopped speaking. The equivalent of breaking the silence with whispers, in DMT, is minute shifts between mobility and immobility. The anorexic 'solution' – an eating disorder, as a substitute for grounding – which devolved into bulimia, caused her bodily self-image to deteriorate. It was as though she moved from the stance of a 'nun', disappearing into anorexia (P0), to the stance of a 'leper', with unbearable presence, picking at her wounds and vomiting (P1).

Over time, a shift occurred in DMT, from the fixated position in the centre of the room to a wall that Anna felt she could lean on; there was a shift from sitting to lying down, with the option of falling asleep (weightedness, gravity, truncal motion, lack of contraction – fulfilling the movement patterns of the parental envelope paradigm). These were minuscule changes, but they highlighted her need for an enclosing envelope and her capability for grounding. It appears that Anna needed a place where she could feel certain her body would not be disturbed, even if she was not on guard. In Anna's case, the split and the lack of integration of the languages were evident: in psychotherapy, she 'vomited' her trauma in a way that was overwhelming, and later fell apart and isolated herself in her room – vertical face-to-face language (P1); in DMT, she developed parental envelope language (P0).

Verbal sharing in psychotherapy alongside bodily and emotional sharing in dance movement therapy

Beth first sought treatment for anorexia at the age of 13. She needed treatment again at 15, for BED (binge eating disorder) and weight gain. She had hospital stays due to depression, suicidal ideation, dysfunction, and orthorexia (obsession with eating healthy food). Beth had suffered physical violence at the hands of her stepbrother and sexual abuse by a cousin of her mother's. Initially, she was alarmed by DMT and frequently complained of boredom, or asked, 'What are we going to do?' In actuality, she took advantage of every moment. Beth had experience with yoga, jazz, and ballet. In our sessions, her pleasure in moving her body was evident, disparate from her willingness to address her eating disorder. Whether through denial or dissociation, she was unable or unwilling to discuss her condition. She was motivated to overcome physical traumas, such as falling off a horse onto her back. She brought her preoccupation with her skin into therapy: the idea of her skin reddening and exposing her. She was concerned with the unequal relationship between us, where she felt she was exploiting me by taking without giving. At home, she was exposed to violence, alcoholism, and drugs during this period. The therapeutic setting was a refuge for her, although she was incapable of relying on an adult and kept herself apart, taking on the role of a 'lone wolf'. In terms of her body, she permitted herself to lean on me by accepting my holding her to descend into a bridge position, and allowed herself to receive when she asked me to place weights on her. Beth demonstrated the ability to accept help on the bodily dimension before the verbal dimension, which is developmentally a later stage.

Beginning therapy for the second time after a hiatus of several years, she entered the remembered room naturally. Sometimes she arrived before I did and I found her waiting for me, but I could not feel angry about her brashness, although the customary practice at this clinic is for the therapist to escort the patient to the therapy room. She moved on from classical music (contained) to modern music (expressive). Beth was reminded of what she had once liked to do in terms of movement. For a moment she tried to do a cartwheel, to stretch her legs out, but then immediately felt self-conscious. She spoke of a loss of flexibility and discomfort with her present weight. She darkened the room, prepared a mattress, lay down facing the floor, and asked me to place weights on her back. Beth struggled to stay in a state of acceptance for long, due to the intense self-hate she experienced. She felt an expression of hope on my part to be a failure of empathy, while she was in pain and crying.

The initial sessions were marked by intense emotionally flooded speech; later, Beth left talking for her psychotherapy and reserved DMT for a bodily experience. She was preoccupied with skin phenomena that exposed what she felt inside, physically and emotionally. She described heat spreading to her arms, while internal motion towards her feet was blocked and they remained frozen. Beth experienced suffering and discomfort with this heat, and with her skin reddening at every movement or touch. She associated these changes with her suicide attempt. I perceived this as an inability to live with an envelope of 'second skin' (Bick, 1968), originally intended to allow her to survive.

Beth asked me to help her stretch her body. She said that when her belly was swollen, a friend would tie a cloth tightly around her abdomen. Stretching also has an aggressive quality; I attempted to help her direct her aggression outward. She said she loved to feel pain in her muscles; she sought deep, powerful touch that would reach to her skeleton.

In the room, she practiced cartwheels and descending into a bridge, taking risks and failing to protect herself. The inverted poses were a response to restlessness, a challenge to the forces of gravity and depression; thus, too, the challenge of doing splits, which to Beth represented the ambition to restore her flexibility. Rising up above the ground, where she was mostly passive, led to active movement: turning a hoop on her hips, sliding on the mats like an ice skater, sexuality and playfulness, and humming to herself in times of trouble, to cradle and soothe herself. Beth seemed to primarily seek contact adapted to her needs, and though she felt guilty for it, she succeeded in asking for what she needed. The touch she had encountered over the course of her life had encompassed physical violence and sexual assault. Beth's mother struggled to contain her children's needs, and lacked the strength to set boundaries for them or to protect them from competing for her attention, from themselves, or from the problematic men of the family. Beth came to the therapy room on her own, and arranged her own space in the room. She had learned that if she did not do so, there would be no space for her; at home, she had no space of her own. She had learned to hold herself prematurely, in the absence of a parental envelope. The touch she requested involved pain, to a certain extent; it is my hope that it was also cushioning, enclosing, healing, safe, consistent, and adapted to her needs, enabling grounding and stabilisation in more secure ground. Beth consciously associated her anxiety and depression with her weight, but, as noted, my understanding is that they derived from the absence of a safe protective envelope in her world. During the period of her treatment, her ability to verbally conceptualise her needs developed and expanded in psychotherapy, paralleling the development of her ability to dissolve and encounter P0 poles in DMT.

Expansion of the ability to cooperate in dance movement therapy with parental envelope paradigm movement – P0

Gaia, 18, suffered from bulimia with vomiting and laxative use, anxiety, and depression, including suicide attempts. She had been sexually abused by a friend of the family. Born with a motor disorder, Gaia was sent to dance lessons from the age of three. In the studio, she danced day and night; in DMT, she refused to move. Her difficulty moving came to the forefront in a session when she grasped a ball and sat facing me with her legs apart; in that moment, Gaia froze, like an animal immobilised. She explained that she was impeded by the embarrassment and shame that engulfed her whenever she was obliged to discuss her world in emotional terms. However, immobilisation with her legs apart may have brought up a bodily memory of trauma that she did not yet have the words to discuss. Gaia said she would like to lie down on the ball, but did not permit herself to do so. The desires and vitality of her body were defensively blocked. Alongside the struggle to move, for Gaia, as an adolescent with an eating disorder, this incident seemed to involve a more dominant primordial physiological difficulty stemming from sexual abuse. Freezing (stopping) and the split position (straightened, large range) belong to the P1 setting, whereas her wish to lie down on the ball (weightedness) is associated with the P0 setting. The verbal wish for enveloping may have been arrested by the vertical face-to-face paradigm, in view of her sexual abuse.

Gaia said she would not move pointlessly; if she moved it would be in a classic way, and she would not move in a classic way because of her high weight. She believed she could help herself, alone, and ruled out any suggestion from me. She played with a ball containing flakes of silver glitter; waiting for all of the flakes to stop moving, her body also froze in a crouched foetal position. When her discomfort and anxiety intensified, she pulled her shirt away from her body and declared that she would do nothing, because she was afraid that any movement would prevent her from gaining weight for her weekly weighing. She helped me inflate balls, with the ostensibly meaningless task allowing her to be active. She played with a ball: inflated it with her mouth, deflated it by squeezing, over and over, as a pulsating body expanding when it feels good and contracting when it feels bad.

Gaia seemed tired, and I asked her if she wanted to doze; she refused. I then suggested a relaxation exercise, and she agreed. When there was an option that could be turned down, it was easier for her to choose something to accept. The acceptance of 'no' is crucial for girls who have been hurt. Gaia enjoyed the twilight states between sleeping and waking. She said relaxation exercises let her detach, like smoking a cigarette. Connecting to herself seemed to involve threat. She struggled when I gave her space without clear instructions, while also needing help and permission just to be.

Her body, contracted and foetal at first, softened and released over time. At first, she felt more comfortable lying on her abdomen. Later, she was able to lie down for relaxation, prostrated and exposed on her back. During our sessions, she transitioned from a protected foetal position to a more trusting position on her back. She seemed to have moved from a resistant, frozen stance to a more committed and warmer stance – from a vertical face-to-face setting, as a protective shield, to a parental envelope setting. Having been born with motor difficulties, Gaia had needed to exert great strengths to attain developmental stages such as moving through space, distancing, and standing upright and stable. These resources were challenged again by the trials of adolescence and by sexual abuse. The result was greater difficulty, but this drove her to receive more support, through therapy, which led to completion of the movement paradigm of the parental envelope space.

Cooperation in dance movement therapy on the vertical face-to-face plane – PI

Dana, 15, suffered from anorexia. Due to financial distress, her family had to leave their home without a stable alternative. The parents were consumed with physical and emotional survival. The family's eldest child, Dana practiced circus arts, excelled at school, and was opinionated and belligerent. She had been sexually assaulted by a respected adult in her community. Dana was a proud girl who kept her distance. From the first session, she stood in the same spot, leaning against the wall. It took hard work to get her to move from leaning against the wall to a more trusting stance, and develop the ability to lean on me emotionally. It was a challenge to soften her position without provoking her rage. Dana came to our relationship from a hostile and suspicious standpoint, resisting and belittling, sarcastic and blunt, and demanded to do whatever she wanted. She was extremely underweight, raising anxiety that her life was at risk, so that it was essential to watch over her. The urge to move drove her to distraction. She would seem to assent to lying down, but the moment she lay on the mat her legs swung over her head and she turned over to stand on her feet again, like a rubber doll.

She was overly flexible, and showed virtuosic abilities even while underweight; her performance made me anxious that she would faint or break. It was hard to stop her. Dana's body was skilled and she was in control, skipping from one to another of the extreme positions she was familiar with. She resisted the therapeutic goal of sensing herself in interim states, with a different quality of movement. She experienced therapy as an attempt to analyse, exploit, and use her – to get something out of her. Guidance was experienced as humiliation. I formed an agreement with her that she could do as she wished for a limited period, in a way that safeguarded her body. She had not practiced circus arts for a year, and she was afraid she might have lost her courage and flexibility. Dana would go into a handstand and cross the room walking on her hands. She explained that her love of exercise was not aimed at losing weight. The permission to move allowed a transition from her hostile, distant stance to a softer and smiling attitude, but there was no deep impact on the relationship. Movement in the vertical face-to-face space appeared to serve as a defence against connection. Hostility was the point of origin; the warming attained was not internalised.

Little by little, Dana responded to slightly different movement: strengthening her muscles against her excessive flexibility, and permitting herself to play and to experience relaxation exercises. Outwardly, even when enjoying herself, she spoke derisively and destructively, saying this was childish and stupid. For my part, I fought for every shred of health. Aware that she was motivated by fear, Dana asked to see adult chronic anorexics, so that she could choose to heal based on being frightened. Her stance close to the wall (upright, straightened, counter to gravity) can be viewed as dominance of the face-to-face setting (P1) – an experience of immobilisation and paralysis, a fear of life. Dana could budge from the wall to exercise, but she struggled to move in a way that would express her feelings or to encounter herself. She asked for ten minutes to do as she pleased, and then to leave. Jumping on a trampoline was freeing for her, but she could jump without me. She thought that when she reached her target weight, DMT – a place to move and gain release – would be taken away from her, until she obtained permission to engage in real training. She expressed a wish to be nourished through a feeding tube forever: 'If only I could train and go outside like this'. Sometimes she calmed while playing elastics, squash, or cat's cradle, but she devalued these moments, with no inner permission to lean, or to be little, in need, and nourished. In the course of her stay, when other girls teased her she did not ask for help, repeating a pattern of lack of trust in adults to help and protect her.

Over time, her hostile attitude softened and her mood lifted. She showed pleasure, release, and a renewed vitality. She asked to listen to music that represented a return to the language of her mother's home, which had let her down. The transference relationship reflected a threat of falling apart and difficulty trusting the world of adults. Dana's actual home and family had broken down when she was a child, and her body went to pieces when she was sexually assaulted. In adolescence, she built up an armour as a gymnast. When that was insufficient she developed an eating disorder, responding to her experience of trauma. Dana was self-contained, proud, and belligerent, calling in a language of her own for nurturance and protection from significant others in her life. In the crisis of continuity in her life, she was emphatic about demonstrating that she was not leaning or dissolving into self-experience in a parental envelope setting. Dana's case illustrates premature maturation of the vertical face-to-face setting. This pathology forms in the absence of appropriate development from the parental envelope paradigm to the vertical face-to-face paradigm.

Transitionality between P0 and P1 – Between vertical grounding and face-to-face grounding

Helen was in therapy for about a year. An emotional bond formed between us from the earliest sessions, progressively deepening, so that it could be referred to as love transference. Helen was a 17-year-old girl with a troubled background who touched my heart. She had undergone psychiatric hospitalisation due to depression and suicidal ideation, and suffered from anorexia. Brutally raped in the past, she had not shared this fact with anyone. During her hospital stay, flashbacks of earlier sexual abuse began to surface. Helen had fallen in love with a woman and would run away from home to be with her, although she too abused her, re-victimising her. She was in therapy in various periods, and was able to accept help in different ways: a period of sleep, of verbal discourse, of bodily movement, and there were times when she would draw. In all of these phases, she gave expression to two voices: a despairing voice and an optimistic voice, one seeking exposure and one shutting down. Alongside feelings of self-hate and guilt, and perceptions of herself as a whore, fat, and better off dead, there were moments of hope, curiosity about the future, a wish for marriage and children and a career, and things she loved; if she was going to live, she wanted to be healthy. These parts were split off and detached, until they came into conflict.

When she was depressed and exhausted, or overwhelmed after psychotherapy, DMT provided a place to rest and relax. She responded to relaxation exercises, and later wanted to sleep; she fell asleep feeling guilty towards the therapist. In psychotherapy, she revealed a real-life abusive relationship, which was reported to her parents; she became extremely upset. She felt she needed a shower or medication to calm down, not DMT. While she felt anger at being guarded, she enjoyed being enveloped. Alongside her wish to repress, she spoke about her relationship with a woman, from which she was in the process of extricating herself, which involved sex, violence, and drugs. It was essential for her to hear from me that she had sought a connection (a parental envelope), and not what she had found – an abusive, exploitative, harmful bond. Together, we differentiated the good things the relationship had given her from the bad. Her partner understood her, calmed her; she loved to go to the beach with her and ride bicycles together at sunset. She was sorry to have spoken about her. Split between bad and good herself, she struggled to see the bad parts of the relationship. She needed recognition for the good parts – to have me with her in that impossible place.

In her body, Helen suffered incessant tension in the back of her neck. She was able to enjoy relaxation exercises, despite her fear that she was contagious; she responded to a bond where she was protected and the boundaries were defined and known. Signs of self-injury to her body were noticeable. Her hands grasped her arms tightly in an attempt to contain the emotional pain, and to be able to feel. Many times I held on to her hands to keep her from hurting herself. I padded her surroundings with mattresses. The moment when she detached was visible in her eyes. During flashbacks, she would slam her elbow, fist, or head into the wall; she said it stopped her from 'traveling', her name for the flashback episodes.

She responded to work on expressing aggression without hurting herself – hitting a roly-poly doll, throwing a ball hard, acting out a temper-tantrum. I worked with her on enhancing her ability to defend herself, not freezing, setting boundaries, and building a new boundary, an envelope for her violated body. She was preoccupied with pent-up weeping, a desire to cry and feel relief, and the difficulty of doing so in the presence of others. She added piercings to her body, writing on herself what she could not tell. She was deeply taken with the scars on her skin – the testament to her history written on her skin – in fear that it might remain, but also that it might be erased. Helen had the capability to express herself and share her story authentically. In a pose where she bent forward, she said the position was unpleasant because it 'made [her] butt feel open'. A foetal position meant to be protective had failed to protect her when she was raped. She found it hard to vocalise, as she had been forbidden to make a sound. From the foetal position, she sent out a hand, as a desperate call for help.

Over time, Helen felt she could and wanted to dance her story. She asked me not to watch, chose music, and danced. She taught me her language: if she was sitting on the floor, that meant it was a bad day when she wanted to die. If she stood up and said, 'It'll be OK', she was aiming for an optimistic mantra but wasn't connected to it yet. She asked me to adopt her; she said she loved me. Gradually, although she always protected me from her anger, she also expressed anger towards me; she said she was wasting my time, and accusingly said I too would report her if she shared her experiences with me. Over and over again, she felt she was left alone and defenceless. She needed my constant support to continue to believe in the process – to believe that while therapy would not change the past, her wound would stop bleeding and running her life. Through a young cousin she cared for, she seemed to care for her inner small child and reconnect with her; mischievous, playful behaviour and enjoyment slowly emerged.

Therapy that began with cooperation in P1 language, without trust building, and could not reach secure and grounded enveloping in the transition to P0 language

Vera, 15 years old, suffered from anorexia, depression, and post-traumatic stress disorder, against a difficult background composed of sexual abuse as well as a childhood spent in a region where severe security-related tensions and threats were commonplace. In our introductory session she was upset; without testing the relationship, she stated she was irritated, asked for a punching bag, and began to hit it. This was an intense encounter for such an early stage in the relationship, and challenged me as a therapist to decide how much to allow and how much to limit and protect. Diving into physical expressiveness in this way (forceful, ballistic – aggressive P1) without building trust was an expression of the complexities that would continue to be inherent in being beneficial and effective for her. At the community centre in the town where she lived, there was a punching bag outside, but Vera avoided using it because she only felt safe in the indoor bomb shelter. She described a continual and incessant state of tension and nervousness that she kept hidden inside because she felt it was an imposition in relationships. The physical expression of her suffering, which she brought to therapy detached from our relationship, made it feel as a burden, not for the weight of her trauma but by the feeling that she could not be helped, despite her cries for rescue.

In reality, the tangible threats of an unstable security situation persisted; at the same time, Vera remained exposed to the person who had abused her. Content was described through hints, while something remained disconnected. Vera often spoke with me on days when we did not have a session scheduled, describing her distress and seeking attention. She drew me in; it was impossible not to respond to her, but these encounters were ineffective. She struggled to be in a bodily experience for long. She shifted between movements of unloading, of strengthening the bodily container, and of releasing tensions and calming down. Sometimes she expressed discomfort and spoke of dizziness, nausea, and pain. Due to the trauma, she said, her body was like that of an old woman. She was afraid to sleep in the dark. When she lay on her back in therapy, the experience of exposure grew more powerful, and she clenched and tightened her knees together to defend herself. The most frequent theme in her sessions was that she said she felt nothing; conversely, she appeared to be feeling too much. She moved between detachment and unbearable emotional flooding. When she described pressure in her chest, the act of repeatedly throwing balls (at medium strength, in a straight line) created movement within the immobilisation of her body. Vera threw the balls while calling the names of the male figures towards whom she directed her rage. She referred to the stack of balls that piled up as the 'mountain of disgust'.

She expressed despair, devaluation, and ambivalence over the possibility of being helped through movement. Feeling her limbs after exertion, she said she did not want to feel that she had hands. I invited her to relax her upper body after a stressful weekend; she asked what the point of release was if she would only grow tense again. Vera said she didn't deserve to drink or eat. When she felt dizzy and I suggested resting her head on the wall, she replied that she would bash it against the wall. At a moment when she was able to deepen her breathing, she said she didn't like to breathe. At other times, she said that everyone hated her and that she felt she wanted to die. Dramatic words such as 'horror' were spoken with a smile, drawing us closer together and simultaneously pushing us apart. Vera had little faith that she could be helped and felt she did not have the strength for the process, but at the same time she gave herself over to it, was eager to please, and carried out any suggestion. She didn't know how to refuse, she explained, and preferred to go with the flow. In this way, the trauma was recreated within the relationship.

She had kept the horror locked away inside her for many years, maintaining the outward appearance that everything was fine, and no-one around her had raised any doubt. An image of 'petrification' came up during the sessions, and we thought together about ways to dissolve it. To Vera, the weak point was her legs, where her paralysis began when she was anxious. She moved and warmed her feet, and a memory emerged from a visit overseas, when her feet felt petrified while riding a scooter – frozen solid, until she accelerated and felt something, and then grew dizzy. She described the precision she needed in order for it to become possible to come into contact with her trauma. She described squeezing her muscles and holding, even in peripheral body parts – her eyes, her feet; we defined this during our sessions as part of a freeze response, and attempted to also spark fight and flight reactions, adding in more parts of the body to attain vitality and pulsing, in contrast to petrification, dying, and, detachment.

There were moments of hope, such as when she told me she had tried to work on her back using a ball, in the bomb shelter. The life story of a girl who had not been seen was interwoven with the traumas of sexual abuse and with the security threats that averted calm to create an envelope that was perforated, convoluted, and difficult to detangle. The eating disorder roused Vera's mother to nourish her and to be the parental envelope for her that she so craved. But when this defence softened and the sexual trauma was more exposed, the parental envelope grew tattered again. Vera was left confused and confusing, once again, recreating a relationship where she could not experience, be aware of, or express herself, either in vertical face-to-face language or in parental envelope language (both paradigms had not matured, and it was impossible to move between them), to herself or to others, in grounded form; not yet. The punch – the ballistic movement at the root of emergence from the parental envelope space to the vertical face-to-face space, the wish she expressed in our first encounter – had not yet ripened.

Discussion

Shahar-Levy (2005) used the emotional movement languages of the parental envelope setting and the vertical face-to-face setting to describe a developmental process through which an organic integration of both languages emerges. In cases where this integration is absent, the patient is held by the therapist in the parental envelope language space (P0), like an infant held by a parent – dependent, passive, collapsing into an oral stance. In cases where the vertical face-to-face language is more salient, the aggression early in therapy is defensive, in contrast to organic aggression. Transitionality is the essence: when parental envelope language can be integrated with vertical face-to-face language, the girl's own envelope thickens, and she gains enhanced ability to resist gravity and fully hatch in the language of bioenergetic analysis, deepening and expansion of vitality in the adolescent girl (self-awareness, self-possession, and self-expression) is interwoven with her capacity for grounding within herself and relational grounding.

The eating disorder itself is a form of self-holding, a substitute for grounding. In anorexia, the avoidance of eating sometimes grants a sense of cohesion. The sensation of hunger seems to collect and tighten the body, making it elongated and narrow, as a substitute for organic verticality. In bulimia, eating and vomiting create an alternative motion in the digestive tract to the vertical up-and-down movement. The grounding that emerges from sexual abuse is traumatic. There is an experience of the ground falling out from underneath oneself, in a deep sense, on the vertical plane and the horizontal plane, as illustrated by the various clinical cases. Beyond the theories presented earlier regarding the ability to be grounded in the vertical plane, into the self, as well as in the horizontal plane in relation to another, and to integrate parental envelope language with vertical face-to-face language, it is important to differentiate the immobility (P0) of paralysis, anxiety, freezing, and rigidity from the movement of soft responsiveness and dissolving, which is made possible through the holding of a present other; the lack of movement, as in the rigid sitting position Anna adopted at first, versus the dissolving prone position of Gaia.

It is also essential to differentiate resistance in the form of avoidance, due to the difficulty of coping with the process, from resistance arising from the ability to refuse, to say no and protect oneself; this quality was often missing in the patients and in their close environment when the sexual abuse and its exposure occurred. Processing trauma requires time, to allow the movement and transition between the poles required for the healing process. Verbal psychotherapy and DMT speak different languages. Therapy aimed at forging a continuity of being between childhood, traumas experienced during life, and the present in adolescence can take various forms. If the process leads to self-awareness and self-possession, to self-experience and self-expression, it has served its purpose.

In DMT, many of the adolescent girls brought up a fear of connecting to themselves and experiencing their bodies if they permitted themselves inward movement, as in breathing, or outward movement in space. It is important to understand that those who move compulsively are on the same axis of dissociation and detachment. Heightened movement with compulsive qualities plays a similar role to lack of movement and immobility, in the sense of the inability to feel the self and the body. In the same way, on the continuum from silence to flooding, girls who share content or expose their bodies in inappropriate ways need protection and help with modulation; they need to be defended, just as the silent girl needs acceptance and encouragement to express herself.

The therapies presented here evoke a theme of self-reliance and difficulty leaning on others. It was essential to most of the girls who had suffered sexual abuse and developed an eating disorder to first build trust, while remaining passive and being held by another. During the course of therapy, they learned to relax their body, breathe and expand on the inside, and exist more fully in a safe and protected space. This is the prerequisite for them to stand on their own, steady and grounded in a reality that has hurt and wounded them. Coping in this way, once they have a stronger and more resilient container, enables them to process and possibly unload some of their burdens within a relationship with another person. In other words, the therapies paint a picture of blocked transitionality between the two modes of connection, or dominance of one relational mode over another. Usually it was the face-to-face setting, the protective shield, that failed to hold, as it was built on the foundation of a parental envelope setting that had not matured – that was lacking, perforated, or confusing. In effective therapy, a process of completion of the poles begins to form: first, the parental envelope, from which the full vertical face-to-face stance can grow.

Many of the themes described were common to patients with eating disorders as well as to patients who had suffered sexual abuse. Despite the commonalities and similarities, the sources of their behaviours may differ. Thus, the tendency towards self-reliance and giving up human objects may arise from sexual trauma in girls with an eating disorder, but may also stem from giving up a human subject, as a result of developmental trauma and object relations. Self-injury, common among both girls with eating disorders and girls who have been sexually abused, is a secondary skin function. This is an envelope that recreates the sexual abuse: perforated and easily penetrated; or an alternative defensive envelope signalling 'no entry', in anorexia.

Conclusion and thoughts for the future

Of 25 cases where both an eating disorder and sexual abuse were present, 14 – more than half – showed change during and through DMT. This is a positive and indeed surprising finding, in view of my own experience as a dance-movement therapist for this segment of patients, which has been accompanied by no small share of frustration, helplessness, and pain. Of the cases I examined, to the extent known during treatment, there were 12 instances of one-time sexual assault, 9 cases of prolonged sexual abuse, 4 cases of significant developmental trauma or injury, and 7 instances of sexual abuse within the family. Of the 25 cases, 4 patients' parents were divorced; 6 had a sibling with an eating disorder; 3 had a sibling with a physical illness; 2 had a sibling with a mental illness; and 4 had a twin.

This was not a statistically reliable quantitative study. It must be taken into account that some cases may not have been identified as involving sexual abuse at the time, and that there were different grades of sexual abuse among the patients. Further, it is essential to take note of the difference between one traumatic event and prolonged trauma, and to differentiate trauma outside and within the family; it is also important when and at what stage the trauma occurred, and whether significant developmental trauma was present. These variations have a substantial impact on the ability of the adolescent and her surroundings to cope with trauma and its consequences. The homes where the girls grew up are similarly significant. In families that experienced divorce or the dissolution of a partnership, there was often an impact on the capacity for parental containment (a collapsing, unreliable parental envelope). In homes where the adolescent has a twin, or a sibling also suffering from an eating disorder or another physical or emotional disorder, resources for coping may be in short supply. Parents' biographies are also meaningful – whether they have suffered traumatic events themselves, including sexual trauma. All of these factors affect the extent of resources available to cope with the sexual trauma and eating disorder of the adolescent herself. There are other variables too, such as the quality of the relationship between the adolescent and her parents, attachment styles, and various disorders and symptoms that can affect an eating disorder as well as sexual trauma – anxiety, obsessive-compulsive disorder, depression, suicidality, post-traumatic stress disorder, self-injury, dissociation, fainting, detachment, attention deficit hyperactivity disorder, modulation issues, rage attacks, impulsiveness, social difficulties, shunning – all of these are crucial to the healing process, as well as influencing the way adolescent girls make use of DMT.

Beyond the findings and the discussion up to this point, there are directions for future thought worthy of further study. It is vital to learn more about the different patterns that become possible in individual DMT, as opposed to group sessions. The work possible in two concurrent therapies could also be studied more deeply, to understand when this practice may be contraindicated. Further, it would be interesting to gain greater understanding of the variance and effectiveness of DMT in comparison to physical education classes. Exercise is crucial to the adolescents for the purpose of weight loss, while also offering additional benefits of discharge that patients may struggle with in therapy that offers a chance for self-expression.

The most essential issue is: which should be treated first, the eating disorder or the sexual abuse? Or should treatment be concurrent? Should the answer to these questions depend on the individual case, or is there a general principle that should apply?

Some patients, after their eating-disorder symptoms had stabilised, were cared for in a setting dedicated to treating sexual abuse, where they mostly met girls suffering from eating disorders.

References

Bick, E. (1968). The experience of the skin in early object relations. *The International Journal of Psychoanalysis, 49,* 484–486.

Lowen, A. (1976). *Bioenergetics: The revolutionary therapy that uses the language of the body to heal the problems of the mind.* London: Penguin Books.

Shahar-Levy, Y. (2005). Tipology of emotive movement. *Dialogues: Journal of Clinical Psychology Israel, S*(3) 1–6 (in Hebrew).

Part III

Dance/Movement Therapy with Adults

Dance/Movement Therapy with Adults

Chapter 5

Focused Therapy for Victims of Sexual Trauma in a Psychiatric Ward

Sigal Nahor Michael and Ariela Lev Rosenblum

Introduction

This chapter addresses the use of Dance-Movement therapy with victims of childhood sexual trauma requiring short-term hospitalisation in a psychiatric ward as adult women. The chapter describes their unique difficulties during hospitalisation, the challenge of working with the abused body, and the common mind-body expressions among them. The various case descriptions describe representations of the echoes of sexual abuse and ways of coping with them. The chapter proposes Dance-Movement therapy as a process that can enable connection to the hurting, rejected, and disconnected body; allowing means of expression for experiences otherwise unexpressed; awakening the body's strengths; and helping victims experience a different presence and liveliness with themselves and with others. These women are hospitalised at times of crisis when they are emotionally overwhelmed and experience an urge for self-injury. Their detachment, dissociative condition, desire for nullification, and desire to die increase. Treatment during these complex situations invites patients to meet the painful and affected body from the past in the present, and to find ways to bring about relaxation in physical-emotional memories, trauma records, and their effects.

During the time I worked with survivors, I found myself repeatedly dreaming the same dream; and in my dream, I travel through time, through large interchanges, trying to return to the past through the traffic on the road. I travel to the next interchange to retrace my steps and twists and turns to reach what was and has been experienced. As time passes, I search for the exact location, the correct exit, the way that will mark my direction.

As in the dream, also in the therapeutic process, we suggest that a therapist should search together with a patient for the 'interchange' that will allow for a 'different exit'. As Levine (1997) wrote, the therapist should start a flow in the stagnated movement and create opportunities for changes in the perception of the body and self. Despite victims' shared trauma characteristics, there is a need to find their unique way, one that will allow them to begin and rethink the body, befriend it, and rely on it when needed.

DOI: 10.4324/9781003309048-9

Focused therapy for sexual trauma victims

In the open psychiatric ward at Israel's Ziv Medical Center, men and women experiencing various mental difficulties, disorders, life crises, and challenges are treated. Hospitalisation is required after self-injury, deep depression, or suicidal situations in order to safeguard patients' lives and then patients gain impulse control. Hospitalisation greatly challenges victims of sexual trauma and produces re-experiences of the trauma. Patients must reside in a mixed ward that accommodates men and women and tolerate impaired autonomy and decision-making regarding the daily schedule, reduced personal space, sleeping in a room with other women, and daily interactions with other patients and staff. A short-term intervention model was initiated in the hospital to provide a dedicated and specially tailored programme for victims of sexual trauma. The main guidelines of the intervention are a 3-week hospitalisation to gain self-regulation, stabilise symptoms, and gain a psychoeducational understanding of the source of the symptoms, in order to continue community-based therapy. During hospitalisation, in addition to various group therapy sessions, each patient receives two different individual treatments: verbal, art, or movement therapy. Each treatment is provided twice a week, closely aided by a social worker and psychiatric treatment.[1]

Because the hospitalisation is short-term and the treatment occurs when the emotional storm is acute, in this chapter we suggest that in Dance-Movement therapy, the therapist should invite the patient to experience grounding (Shuper Engelhard, Pitluk, & Elboim-Gabyzon, 2021): that is, a feeling of stability, being present in the here and now, reducing and controlling symptoms, renewed emotional balance, and body-mind 'thickening of the skin' by strengthening ego forces and the sense of visibility.

Dance movement therapy with survivors of childhood sexual trauma

The territory of the body – an area been intruded on, violated, and harmed – the battlefield of sexual assault cannot be taken for granted as an instrument of therapeutic intervention. Among survivors of sexual trauma, the body can arouse anxiety, rejection, concerns, avoidance, and even resistance. The difficulty of relating to the body is associated with self-perception and body image, which often include rejection of the body, hatred and anger at its 'betrayal', distrust in it, detachment from its feelings, and disregard for its needs (Lowen, 1995). Patients also describe difficulty enduring the presence of others in the same space and other bodies moving around them simultaneously. This, as Levine (1997) put it, is because the threat to the personal and physical space brings the mind-body system to a state of constant arousal and vigilance, which are summoned at the slightest movements in space.

In reference to the place of the body's story in childhood sexual abuse, Herman (1994) wrote that sexual abuse harms the evolving soul, the formation of close relationships, and interpersonal conduct. Abuse produces many physical consequences expressed in the body's position, movement-conduct in interpersonal space, and somatisation. Trauma impairs the perception of the body and self and the ability to engage in emotional and physical intimacy. It can lead to eating disorders and problems in various biological systems such as skin, digestion, and sex.

The confused perception of time and the lack of clarity in perceptions of space, body, and surroundings also characterise victims of childhood sexual trauma in adulthood. Transitions between different periods of life through re-experiences, flashbacks, nightmares, or other parts of personality repeatedly occur for several moments or entire days (Van der Kolk, 2015). The abuse returns and reconstructs itself in different ways. The body that is the battlefield where the assault occurred, which continues to be repeatedly re-experienced, is a threatening and challenging arena.

In sexual assault within close relationships in childhood, the mind deals with what cannot be thought of through fragmentation, detachment of parts of the consciousness, parts of the body, and parts of the self – as Gurevich (2018) wrote, a 'survival dissociation' – that leaves a mark of the negative of the traumatic event. The experience appears as floating dream fragments, or floating nightmare tears, in physical symptoms and interpersonal relationships. The long therapeutic process of exposing, witnessing, re-experiencing, and validating passes through merging the split and disconnected parts to create a new integration.

During the brief hospitalisation, rifts will not heal, the whole story will not be told, and integration will be, at best, just beginning. In this situation, therapy will often end just as different puzzle pieces begin to connect, with a momentary view into the representations of the aggressor and the victim, the negative of the trauma and its echoes.

Dance movement therapy allows an understanding of trauma's effects. In addition to the traumatic themes that arise in the body, Dance-Movement therapy allows connection to sources of strength and physical regulation and a process of befriending and reconnecting with the body.

Not all survivors can participate in Dance-Movement group therapy when the group includes women and men. Most are initially reluctant to participate in individual therapy, which focuses on movement and attention to the body. Shaham (2017) referred to non-movement situations that characterise the treatment of patients who have Post-traumatic stress disorder (PTSD). A case of non-movement presents itself as a difficulty in arising from the holding and shielding chair into the space of the room and span of movement. Non-movement indicates a need to expand the perception of motion and how to get it started. These situations are evident among women with complex PTSD, which is differentiated from PTSD in the continuation of the assault and its existence within a relationship, primarily when the assault occurs in early childhood, when the mind and soul are still developing (Herman, 1994).

The case descriptions in this chapter describe that alongside the difficulties, compliance with relating to the body in the healing process allows an opening to emerge and enables an exit from patterns established as a result of trauma. In my experience, even with patients who hated their body and initially resisted even feeling it, one can see upon their return to a second or third hospitalisation a change in trust and a willingness to think about themselves and their bodies differently. What follows are vignettes from treatments; these demonstrate the role of the therapist who tries to hold different parts of the treatment of trauma, anchor them in the body and the word, and give them meaning and continuity within a relationship, in a short time and when the therapy objectives are focused.

Focusing on body sensations to identify dissociative attack

> *The only way for the body to survive the pain of the assaults I went through was not to feel at all.*

One way for the mind and body to copy with an assault is to detach from sensation – to reach a point where one cannot feel one's body or think about it. This condition may be accompanied by a loss of sensation in the skin (Levine, 1997) or a numbness of the body's sensations (Lowen, 1995).

Nanette, who has a large build and is obese, arrived at the ward after long-term physical neglect. She had long kept to herself in her home and avoided contact with the outside world; she did not shower and had an unpleasant body odour. Not entirely consciously, she instigated rejection from her environment and prevented people from approaching her. Hospitalised with depression and a desire to no longer live, she responded slowly to attempts to communicate with her, her speech had a low tone and volume, she conversed little, and her answers resolved to 'I don't know'. She sat fully reclining in the chair, her hands resting helplessly, with almost no movement, and only a playful little smile peeked for a moment. Her entire physical presence conveyed the message 'Don't touch me and don't come near me', but something about her little smile drew me to find out what was hidden under the layers she was wearing.

Nanette suffered from dissociative episodes in which she would harm herself. The focus of her therapy process was preliminary identification of attacks to gain control over them. In the first few sessions, I tried to guide her to listen to the feelings of her body inside the room, such as heat or coolness, but at first she felt nothing. She said that during dissociation, she re-experienced her trauma, and her way of stopping it was with sharp pain, cutting her hands or lacerating her legs. Nanette said that that was the only pain strong enough to return her to reality. Other sensory stimuli with which she learned to ground herself and stop the dissociation, like the smell of lemon, a painting of a beloved artist, or even ice in her hand, didn't help. Nanette added that she had felt no pain even during a car accident in which she was involved. Despite the exterior appearance that prompted distancing from her, I felt an inner warmth towards her in our encounters in the room, which signalled to me that she also has tenderness and pleasantness.

To produce a sensory, physical grounding, an experience of physical presence here and now, we looked at the therapy process for the sensory components experienced as safe and pleasant for her. Levine (1997), in the somatic experi-ence approach, talked about the importance of connecting to the 'sense of sens-ing', a feeling that produces tranquility and stable grounding in the present. Nanette spoke of perfumes she liked and of listening to reggae music because of the melodies and rhythms. After establishing positive body sensations as a resource for control and relaxation, we began exploring what triggers disso-ciation and detachment and the physical signs that precede it. Nanette could say that the dissociation was preceded by rapid breathing, but she had trouble stopping and immediately experienced dissociation. She described men's voices as a cause of stress and the evening hours as darkness falls making it more difficult. We sought ways to obscure and prevent the penetration of sensa-tions that stimulate dissociation and to solidify her sensory sheath. Nanette suggested walking around with headphones, listening to reggae music, and turning on the light in her room before dark. These seem like simple methods, but Nanette, who was abused throughout her childhood to the point that she ran away from home, did not internalise a regulating and relaxing parental figure. She needed psychoeducational intervention, sometimes very primary, to solidify her mind-body skin so that it would be less permeable and accessible and to find ways to regulate her emotions.

Later in therapy, Nanette shared that running water triggers strong feel-ings and stress and that she thus avoids showers. We practiced expansion of thought through mental imagery during therapy to other water sources that do not bring on the same sensations and tensions. Nanette said that the sight of a flowing stream calmed her, and she recalled being on vacation with her family at a magical scene on the edge of a stream. We practiced expanding the pleasant body sensation that accompanied this good mem-ory that led to relaxation radiating throughout her body. Peace created in the body serves as a physical resource according to the somatic experience approach (Levine, 1997). Using imagination allowed Nanette to expropri-ate the trapped context created between the sensation of water on the body and the trauma. These are the same 'memory clusters' as in Shahar-Levy (2004), in which a connection was established between sensory, emotional, movement, thought, and interpersonal experience – memory clusters that froze in time because of the trauma and did not continue to flex and develop.

After remaining in the feelings, identifying them, and being able to use them in the present, Nanette described another element that sabotages her relationships with her family: 'I don't speak of what I feel, want, or need. I just act it out', similar to the way it was reconstructed at the beginning of our relationship. She shared that as a child, any emotional expression would make her more vulnerable in the eyes of her surroundings and that therefore, to this day, she does not express emotions.

Nanette seemed to have created dissociations in the feelings of her body, the feeling of emotions, and thinking about them. She followed patterns that helped her survive as a child and maintain her sanity, but today they do not assist her and even make it more difficult for her. At the same time, the option of thinking about her bodily sensations differently was opened before her, alongside the option to use imagination to summon beneficial sensory experiences and expand them as a tool for relaxing and regulating feelings. Van der Kolk (2015) talked about the awareness of the delicate sensations that arise from within the body, introspection, which allows the beginning of attaining 'agency', a term that describes the feeling of a person being in control of his or her own life. According to Van der Kolk, the greater the awareness, the greater the potential to control our lives.

Dissociation from the body and reconnecting

I came out of my body, I floated with the angels who asked me if I wanted to return to earth, they told me it would be difficult, but I chose to return ... I landed like an angel with broken wings.

Disconnecting from body sensations, detachment from the emotions that accompany the act, and disconnecting from the thought of it, are protections the body uses to survive pain. Dissociation allows the soul to avoid humiliation, offense, helplessness, and pain. The experience of depersonalisation enables loss of the sense of self and a sensation as if observing assault from a distance (Van der Kolk, 2015). The victim pays the price for these protections that affect the course of their life, whether in the inability to use the body's sensations to signal the brain to internal and external reality or in the inability to feel present and alive in the body, as described through Nurit's story.

When Nurit entered the room, she took off her shoes and sat on the floor, engulfed in tears. She said that the very thought of the body overwhelms her. She hasn't felt her body in years, as if it's activated with 'copy-paste' and not under her control. Since the age of seven, when she disconnected from her body and froze so as not to feel it, she can't go back to feeling it again. Nurit said that only when riding a motorcycle does she feel physically alive. The jolting and lurching, the movement of the pelvis and thighs, the advancement through space, and the wind in her face allow her to feel so. I invited Nurit to try the body position on a motorcycle, but she was not ready to experience a similar movement within the room. She said that it immediately triggered the re-experiencing of the abuse. It seemed at first that moving her body in my presence was impossible for her. Almost every position or movement aroused memories of the abuse or thoughts of her relationship with her brother and mother. She said that her mother had always treated her with criticism and rejection. She was disgusted with her and said that Nurit arouses lust in men. Thus, the critical view was internalised, creating unbearable guilt, and Nurit could not think of her body in any other way. She described difficulty separating what happens around her from herself and her memories. She shared that in order to avoid hearing and feeling her reality as a child, she invented memory games to divert her attention from what was happening: 'I taught myself too well to disconnect, and now it is turned against me'.

Although Nurit was ashamed of her body and its presence, she also wanted to work with it in therapy because of an inner feeling that that is where the key lies. We tried together to look for a way in which she could move, and at Nurit's request, we found an exercise that, by shaking her pelvis while lying on her back on a mattress, allows the release of the pent-up energy in the body. This time, Nurit asked to move in my presence as I watched. Perhaps because it's a predetermined movement, a repetitive one, already practiced at home; maybe because she wanted me as a witness. I sat on the floor at some distance from her, witnessing her process and allowing my body to resonate with her from inside (Fishman, 2016). Nurit lay on her back, moving her pelvis back and forth, up and down, and I couldn't help but envision the act of abuse and feel waves of sexual arousal in my lower abdomen. During the experience, Nurit talked about the body's position during the assault. For moments, it was unclear whether she was dissociating, which caused me to feel alarmed, or concentrating on her movements and what they brought up in her. I remained sitting next to her, holding inside me the panic and the consent to witness her moving her body in a way related to the abuse she had suffered.

It seemed as if Nurit was trying to pass something on to me from what she had experienced in order to convey what couldn't be said. Seligman (2016) argued: 'The event does not articulate, and therefore does not become a memory that can be told. Even if there are words that outline the event, they are never enough. The awareness is missing, the historical continuum, the context. At the same time, the trauma does not leave the victim alone and seeks to reach an end, to register, to be recognised or be delivered to another' (p. 143). Experiencing the movement created a relative relaxation of the physical tension and allowed the emotions hidden in the body to surface.

Nurit spoke of feelings of shame and guilt that were immediately linked to abuse, the humiliation of the feeling that her soul was taken from within her upon penetration, and that she was left empty: 'I imagined the assailant collecting my little soul and keeping it in a box'. These words made me feel guilty for letting her dive into the depths of her memory and be hurt again. And yet it seemed that my mere presence near her, even without words, only my reassuring gaze, my willingness to remain with her in the areas of trauma and to experience it both in my body and in my memories, enabled partial modulation. As Seligman (2016) wrote, 'in the process of mutual influence, in which the subjectivity of the therapist and that of the patient meet, affect each other and influence one another, the therapist involuntarily penetrates and is penetrated, as an integral part of the therapeutic process' (p. 145).

Nurit arrived at the next session experiencing severe back pain and could not move her pelvis. I felt a contraction in my diaphragm that directed me to a blockage in my breathing. I suggested lying on a mattress, practicing meditation, and breathing into the pain. According to Fishman (2016), through the process of somatic counter transfer, the dance therapist facilitates the self-development of a client when the process has been blocked or interrupted. It is essential that the therapist be open to one's inner sensations and feelings and be aware of what is familiar in one's own movement. Understanding, acknowledging, and interpreting the experience of movement sensing and how movement makes sense are functions inherent to the therapeutic processes. At this point, with the expansion of the breathing, we added the experience of extracting air and sound taken from the bioenergy analysis, allowing the release of a 'body armour' (Reich, 1972) created to protect the tender soul and over the years becoming a barrier and blockage. Lowen (1995), following Reich, talked about avoiding emotions that affect the depth of breathing, which reduces vitality and leads to long-term chronic muscular tension.

This experience raised, as Nurit put it, 'the sigh that I haven't sighed in a long time', and she then shared that it was forbidden to sigh and complain about life at home. Various body sounds made her brother feel disgusted. Thus, she avoids them and breathes in a limited way so that no sound is heard. Nurit spoke of the heavy load on her back and shoulders and the effort to stay focused on the present. We added physical experiences to release the stiffness and tensions. According to the Emotorics psychodiagnostic tool, the ability to transition between opposing poles within the movement experience is the way to reach balance and feel present and vital (Shahar-Levy, 2004). I moved between contraction and relaxation with her, stretching, straightening, and expanding to curving, contracting, and reduction. With the calming of the physical aspects, she could be present with her body and its movements, without judgment or criticism. During therapy, the way to return to the physical sensation and vitality was opened – the way to beneficial movement for her own body and to be present in her own body with a soft, non-judgmental, or critical gaze.

Body hatred and self-injury

I never have a beginning and never have an end.

Many victims of sexual abuse experience self-loathing: hatred for the body that betrayed and a desire to punish it, both for its betrayal and as part of the aggressor components implanted in the soul as 'foreign implants', a term established by Ferenczi (1995, p. 118). The associated self-injuries are not only used for punishment. Sometimes they are used to resurface from dissociation, to reduce emotional pain through the sight of blood and the feeling of bodily pain, or during a dissociative state as if re-experiencing the abuse in a kind of compulsive repetition.

Ora entered the room and sat down, making no eye contact, occasionally peeking in my direction. She moved to sit on the floor and said that she felt safe this way and that 'I don't deserve to sit at the same height as other people'. I debated whether to sit on the floor as well, which I sometimes do with patients in order to be on the same eye level and meet their gaze, but I felt that Ora was asking for herself at this point, the current location in the room and the relationship. Ora shared that she always hides behind doors so that people won't be able to come in and see her. She responded with a jump to every sound or noise but managed to calm herself down, saying to herself, 'It's okay'.

In the face of her hyperarousal and vigilance, I felt my space of movement and breathing diminished. I perceived that any fluctuation would make her jump. Ora talked about biting and jaw locking as relieving her stress and enabling her to express a connection of love. She mocked this inefficient behaviour but said that she could keep doing it until she bled, especially in dissociative situations and sometimes consciously. Later, she differentiated between dissociation and flashback. She described an ability to detect an impending dissociation, characterised by weakness and dizziness, but not knowing how to identify the arrival of a flashback. In a flashback, she returns to her childhood, which can last many hours. She is unaware of the passage of time, and only when looking at her watch again does she realises that she was in a dissociative state. Her roommates in the ward told her that she hits herself, and she said she feels as though she is suffocating, and that sometimes she grabs herself around the neck – that she re-experiences the events done to her as a child and during the dissociation.

As she spoke in the treatment room, she occasionally fell into thought or disconnection; she was not always present with me; and when I said her name, she smiled and returned to me. She seemed to take a kind of pleasure from the alarm stirring up in me and from keeping indirect control over me with her descriptions of helplessness when I became helpless in response to her. During our first meeting, one of the matrices written about by Davies and Frawley (1994) was manifested in the switch between abuser and helpless victim. As we discussed regaining control, it was evident that she was becoming more stressed: she began to breathe quickly, and her leg became numb. Attempts to practice grounding using her legs were met with the response 'I hate my legs, they're ugly'. A suggestion to touch her legs with her hands to restore feeling was met with the response 'I am disgusted by any kind of touch, including my own'. With close guidance, she was ready to experience briefly but held on to her helplessness and the desire to only talk, not to listen to her body, or to think about her body that had been harmed on so many levels.

Ora found it challenging to relate to her body directly, but, using a projective instrument, she could think about it. She showed me a drawing: 'I drew the falcon flying over the dove, I spread out both their wings and for the dove I also drew tree branches and legs to hold on with'. The drawing expressed her fear and inability to trust, confide in, or rely on others. But she also gave the dove legs to stand on and a branch to do so – grounding. Ora could begin to use imagination and creativity to allow distancing and symbolisation of the experience.

I'm too much for people; no one can hold space for me.

Upon her return to the psychiatric ward for a second time, Ora asked to focus on connecting to reality, to the here and now. We began by exercising by touching one palm to the other. Ora responded with half a smile, saying that she hated feeling her body and hands. I suggested that she should move towards me, place her palms against mine and implement isometric force (implementation of pressure without moving in space) by touching hands and leaning one against the other to give the body a sense of where it ends and to give the energy stored in its implementation (Shahar-Levy, 2004). Ora applied force and said that this is how she feels more present in her body and that this movement does not provoke disgust. Since I knew of her fear and objection to moving in space, I tried to expand the experience by suggesting that she apply force on an object. This idea was met with much hesitation. When Ora said that she hates every movement she makes and does not want to think of herself moving in space, when I said that life itself generates movement anyway, she replied spitefully, 'So I'll stop moving altogether'. Ora seemed to sway between agreeing to accept my offers, trusting me, pushing me away, and making threatening statements hidden behind half a smile. She expressed the internal conflict within her soul and body when she experiences stagnation in the face of life that requires movement, change, and reaction.

To create an 'interchange', I switched to the cognitive channel and explained the importance of searching for grounding techniques and changing the thinking patterns and conduct that do not benefit her. We tried to move to a technique that includes pushing one's feet hard against the floor while sitting on a chair, again using isometric force. When I suggested stomping on the ground, Ora became distressed and, from there, spiralled into dissociation without her or my being able to stop it. She sat huddled on the chair, her palms clenched as though paralysed, protecting her head and body; any sound or voice made her jump; it looked like she was trying to defend herself against external blows. I cringed in terror, witnessing her state, the scene in which I was taking part. I repeated her name, reassuringly saying that she was in the ward, in a safe place, but it was no use. I brought an icepack and held it close to her hands, voicing and foretasting my actions. At first she recoiled from the cold touch, but then she held on to it, calmed down a bit, and managed to get up and go to bed.

During our meeting two days later, we discussed what had happened and what had led to the dissociation. Ora could not describe precisely what caused it: the sound of the legs on the ground, or the movement itself. I felt guilty for hurting her with my suggestion of movement, and I apologised for that; I suggested that she tell me to stop when I am not at one with her needs. But Ora said that she couldn't tell me or anyone else to stop. In retrospect, it was evident that an isometric movement was more available to her, whereas rapid rhythm or release remained threatening and experienced as a loss of control. There was also the relationship component between us; I became the assailant within the initial re-experienced matrix of relationships in the close connection.

Relistening to the body and searching for control

Let the wound heal and learn to live with the scar, even if it opens sometimes.

By this time, Ora knew how to detect the onset of a dissociative episode. She said she felt that her legs were unresponsive. Gradually the detachment spreads throughout her body until it is completely paralysed, and she cannot control it. At the same time, she hears all the swearing and hostile words aimed at her in her head. She said she feels cut off from her legs and has hated them since she was a child; they always froze and allowed others to hurt her: 'I've completely cut myself off, I don't feel any sensation in them, and I don't pay attention to them'. I suggested using the sensation in her legs as a signal for what would come, to get up and walk, pump blood to them before she loses feeling, and thus gain control. But Ora fended off this suggestion with a smile. At the same time, she began to walk around with a notebook of mandalas, filling them out with soothing back-and-forth movements throughout the session, which allowed her to speak and regulate her tension (using the sucking rhythm; Kestenberg-Amighi, Loman, Lewis, & Sossin, 1999).

Leading up to her release, Ora spoke of movement and her body, about her difficulty with her body and all its motions. About me not being attentive to her, and suggesting something difficult for her, grounding using her legs. She could talk about my empathic failure directly to me, without dissociating and without lashing out, and could even specify one particular position of forearms on knees that gives her a feeling of strength, presence, and vitality. She shared that she was exercising in her apartment alone, feeling relaxed and taking out her aggression on a punching bag, imagining someone she wanted to punch.

We continued discussing the aggressive movement as something that allows grounding, releasing contained energy, and excretion of soothing hormones; about the possibility of sublimating the expression of anger and rage. At this point, Ora could begin to think of her body and its movement in the world in a controlled manner, to begin releasing and taking out aggression herself, but not yet in a relationship.

Ora struggled with saying goodbye, said that she felt like she was collapsing from inside, but also spoke of plans for the future. She wanted to set up a therapeutic space for women who were abused. She wanted to use female affinity, creative areas, and the body's wisdom. Ora could imagine herself in the future and as having meaningful accomplishments stemming from internalising what she learned during her stay in the ward. She could hold different parts, benevolent and abusive, in herself and the therapeutic relationship with the option for reconciliation. And, as she put it, 'Let the wound heal and learn to live with the scar, even if it opens sometimes'.

Physical symptoms

I understand my body is talking, but it's hard for me to listen to it.

There are many physical symptoms. The symptom 'speaks' what cannot be thought of, or what the soul lacks words to express. In an early stage of pre-mentalisation, the ability to turn raw experience into symbolic representations that words can describe is missing. Therefore, trauma settles in the body. Shahar-Levy (2004) referred to the mechanism of displacement from the musculoskeletal system to the autonomous system. The autonomous system matures even before the motor system and thus becomes the primary route for expressing excitement. Herman (1994) argued that chronic overstimulation disrupts the normal regulation of physical conditions calmly and consistently, and thus sleep disturbances, eating disorders, aches, and physical symptoms develop. Symptoms can include pain, especially in the abdominal and pelvic areas, a sensation of detachment from different body parts, excessive cleanliness or avoiding showers, low sensory registration or hypersensitivity, problems in the urinary and sexual systems, and arthritis. Dina's story presents the physically symptomatic expression and its role as a substitute for unbearable emotions.

As soon as she entered the room, Dina asked whether it was possible to sit at a distance. She first sat in a chair, and then grew cold, and I offered her a blanket. Upon receiving the blanket, she asked to sit on the beanbag chair. She sat on it, wrapped up, leaning against the wall, and was immediately absorbed with tears. 'I'm not comfortable with my body, everywhere, and I have trouble finding a place where I'm comfortable', she said. It was evident that she was having difficulty breathing and was about to have a panic attack. I felt my breathing grow shallow in response and suggested that we try breathing techniques. Dina refused, withdrew into herself, and began gasping, and I felt the beginning of dizziness. These somatic experiences were described by Ogden (1992) as experiences of somatic countertransference, which is expressed in physical sensations. I was worried that she would hyperventilate and disconnect from me. I suggested that she stand up to improve her breathing and create physical grounding. As Lowen (1995) put it, such grounding strengthens a person's connection to the body and to reality.

Dina stood up and asked to go out and breathe some fresh air. I went out with her, standing some distance from her, giving her some space and feeling that I was losing her before we had even begun. I realised that being in the room was too intimate for her and, thus, difficult; we had to take the journey differently. I suggested taking a short walk together. Walking allowed movement in the extremities and an exit from the freeze mode she entered. It also allowed us to be together, side by side, maintaining a dynamic interpersonal space that she could control, rather than directly face to face, in 'vertical face to face', according to Shahar-Levy (2004).

The ability to be in 'vertical face to face', one opposite the other, is related to fundamental relationship outlines and may threaten those who have experience abuse in a relationship. As we walked, her breathing experienced a lull, and we discussed her experience. Dina was concerned with the question of what sexual abuse is, what body parts are involved, in what way, and whether she had been sexually abused or not. Without knowing the circumstances of her abuse, I reflected the confusion created especially in a little girl and when the abuse occurs in a significant relationship within the family (Ferenczi, 1955). In our discussing the confusion between the language of tenderness and desire, Dina added that another language exists in sexual abuse: that of humiliation. She said that her roommate in the ward told her that it was worth 'jumping into the water' in therapy but that she found it very difficult to talk about her body, to move with or feel it. She said that she knows there are many ways she can learn, but that all the breathing techniques and observing of the body make it more difficult for her. She realises that her body is speaking to her but has difficulty listening to it; she suffers from pain throughout her body that has accompanied her for years, 'not really fibromyalgia, but lots of painful areas'.

Dina spoke of constantly feeling ridiculous as she moved and of feeling dirty. As a child, she would scrub herself with steel wool to remove the dirt that clung to her. Currently, she showers upon every transition from activity to activity or from task to task. She hates perspiring; she feels like she is filthy, and she sweats even more because of the stress. She holds back a lot on going to the bathroom and has trouble letting go and relaxing her muscles to relieve herself. I proposed a physical movement of contraction and relaxation, mainly of the sphincters, while explaining the mind-body mechanism that is activated in constant contraction, about the hyperarousal and constant vigilance when the system is out of balance (Levine, 1997). Over the years, I have found that in situations of hypervigilance, locking the sympathetic system in a state of physical contraction, the instruction to relax is not always available. To release oneself from suspension, one should first move towards contraction to find the opposite pole, and then the movement between contraction and relaxation is possible. Thus, we worked together in contracting and relaxing different body parts: first with the large muscles that activate the hands, legs, and torso; the muscles of the motor system; and later also with the inner muscles, the sphincters.

At our next meeting, Dina sat in an armchair leaning against the door with her head pressing against it. When someone accidentally tried to come in, she pushed the door back with her shoulders and head. I was startled; I felt intrusion into the safe space of the room and a contraction in my diaphragm, and I stopped to clarify the physical sensation with her. Surprisingly, Dina spoke of a good feeling in her body, a sense of control, because she pushed against the door and succeeded. I reinforced the ability to push, and we developed different options of pushing with the hands that allow you to feel body boundaries, strength, and control. The ability to push and repel, not possible during abuse, gives the body a feeling of where it ends and gives it a shell. It enables the use of the life force to protect and express herself and gives her a sense of control over the situation (Shahar-Levy, 2004).

At the next meeting, Dina chose to sit in 'vertical face to face' in a chair closer to me, upright, looking directly at me, and told me about her plans for after her release from the hospital. She said that she had aggressive thoughts towards her father. She asked whether I could stomach her descriptions or whether it would be too overwhelming. Without waiting for a response, she quoted a phrase taken from the holy scriptures, 'to comb his face with iron combs and cut into his flesh', as an expression of her aggressive fantasies. I simultaneously experienced the horror, the thought of what her flesh had been through, and the panic that she might yet attack the assailant in this way. Dina said she knows that she won't act on these thoughts but that when they arise in her, she feels guilty about their very existence. We expanded in conversation about permission to give space to aggressive thoughts of vengeance and destruction without carrying them out, the possibility of expressing anger, and the energy stored in it, both verbally and physically.

Dina shared that she sometimes takes a pen and paper and fills large areas with back-and-forth movements. Kestenberg-Amighi et al. (1999) referred to congenital and acquired rhythms used for soothing, among them the 'back and forth' movement, which constitutes a sucking rhythm whose purpose is to achieve primal regulation. I suggested that she use movements that diverge from the body plane and include direction and strength against a punching bag, but Dina said that doing so would escalate the feeling. It seemed that she needed the relaxation from the back-and-forth movement, even if it resulted in increased muscle tone, and that an outward movement, focused and with force, was not yet available for her. Lowen (1995) wrote about muscle stiffness that leads to joint pain, which holds the anger and fear of it, and argued: 'There is a strong resistance as to the expression of anger towards the abuser. It stems partly from guilt about participating in the sexual act, whether voluntarily or coerced. But the resistance also stems from the fear of the anger that is experienced as a desire to kill' (p. 231).

Turning her attention to breathing, Dina said, 'I always take small, shallow breaths so that no one can hear me; sometimes I feel like I'm not breathing at all'. She said that during panic attacks, she feels numb and lacks control of her extremities. During the meeting, a psychoeducational explanation of the mechanisms of physical response was provided: fight, flight, and freeze, as the body's response to a tangible or internal threat (Levine, 1997). Dina was ready to continue working with the body and to move from her initial contracted state to movements that discharge energy through grounding and experiencing stomping the ground and movements that allow the feeling of strength and intensity (such as running). In Shahar-Levy's (2004) terms, 'powerfulness' refers to the use of force to move forward in life, and 'forcefulness' combines self-expression with strength.

At first Dina was embarrassed, but since we did it together, she allowed herself to explore the movement suggested, which led her to experience a feeling of bodily presence and liveliness. The joint movement in the treatment room enabled interpersonal reverberation, permission to express force, and an experience that she is not alone in the world. Kleinman (2016) described three concepts in the therapeutic relationship of Dance-Movement that facilitate the process: rhythmic coordination (synchronisation) – the ability to be attuned to ourselves and the patient, movement awareness – the ability of a person to feel his or her physical self on an internal and external level, and kinaesthetic movement empathy – the perception of emotional behaviour in another and immediately experiencing it within the body.

After creating stable and safe grounds between us, we could then work on breathing techniques for relaxation to gain self-control during dissociation. This work focuses on prolonging and slowing each breath, especially prolonging the duration of exhalation to prevent hyperventilation and enhance soothing (Lowen, 1995). Daily practice was suggested to be available to her even during a dissociative episode. Upon her release from the ward, she said that she was taking all of these to work on and gain control over her emotions and PTSD so that they wouldn't control her.

The fury trapped in the body

For 20 years, I've just been silent and absorbed or ran away; now I have a lot of fury in me.

Van der Kolk (2015) wrote about the therapeutic approaches that merge 'top to bottom' interventions, activating the social engagement system, and 'bottom-up' interventions, calming physical tensions in the body. Accordingly, breathing exercises, martial arts, drumming, singing, and group dancing based on interpersonal rhythms, physical awareness, and voice or facial expression communication help people leave 'fight or flight' situations and strengthen their ability to sustain relationships.

Lenore, a small, thin, dyed-hair woman who prominently neglected her teeth, sat down as she entered the room with a side turn, her hands enclosing her chest and her legs trembling slightly. Her gaze was sometimes impenetrable and detached and sometimes mocking and irritated. Speaking only in response to questions, without initiative, she was irritated and impatient. She brought a lot of anger about the world, about feeling helpless in the face of authorities. She talked about feeling lonely; she needed someone to support and accompany her but didn't believe that anything or anyone could really help and said that she didn't trust anyone: 'There is no point in bonding or believing that something will change; you are only doing your job anyway'.

She talked of internalised exploitation, criticism, and humiliation: 'I didn't know any better; I thought that's how you behave in a relationship'. She added, defiantly, that she didn't have the strength to think about the past again and that doing so wasn't helping her. She wanted to do something else, but she did not know what. Her leg tremors increased, and since she refused to do any work on breathing, I invited her to a physical discharge of energy. My invitation was accompanied by a psychoeducational explanation about the constant state of stress and vigilance she is in. The stagnant sediment of energy did not dissipate when she could not fight or escape. That energy is trapped in the nervous system, corresponding to the concept of somatic experience (Levine, 1997). Gradually she looked up at me and, for a few moments, was also able to maintain 'vertical face to face' and to sit facing me. Later, she calmed down and could talk more freely. I suggested that she try moving in a manner influenced by her convoluted sitting, emphasising centring, balancing, and achieving control over her body. The movement in the twisted positions and the opposite directionality enabled the insertion of liveliness, a sense of flow in the body, and finding balance and equilibrium. Such movement is a mental challenge, requiring movement across the body midline. It is considered more developed and strengthens the connection between the two lobes of the brain. Visible here, as Marianne Chase put it (as cited in Fishman, 2016), are the modalities of the reference therapy in response to the patient's movement patterns. A movement that allows him or her to feel validation and an inner presence.

When Lenore felt safer, she reported reacting aggressively in many interpersonal situations. She knows that it is inefficient but finds it hard to think about gaining self-control. She said that over the years, she had learned to be angry but that she cannot cry, adding painfully, 'How can it be that a woman like me who's been through so many traumatic events does not cry?' Van der Kolk (2015) argued that 'when patients can carry the physical experiences associated with trauma … They will discover powerful urges within their bodies … That awoke during the trauma but were suppressed to survive. These urges are expressed in subtle movements such as twisting, turning the body … By increasing these movements, the process of reconciling with them begins' (p. 283). It seemed that Lenore began to move the stagnated energy, feel her emotions, and express them.

Nullify, cut or dance with the body

Shahar-Levy (2004) described the use of powerful movement: a movement that musters force and uses the extremities to produce movements that extend into the surroundings. This movement enables the experience of ability and vitality. I bring Darry's story of the tumultuous movement between the urge to die and the urge of life, between the wish to nullify or attack, and the possibility of moving and dancing the pain and the joy. Upon arriving in the ward, Darry was experiencing high levels of anxiety. Entering the room, she looked around as if examining the place. Her head constantly moving in every direction, she resembled a hunted animal. She sat down, her legs trembling, a tremor that occasionally spread to her entire body. She spoke clearly, looking straight at me, but from time to time it seemed that she disengaged or was deep in thought.

Darry shared that she was struggling with her body and its presence. She suffered from anorexia; and with weight gain and returning to her expected weight, she finds it more difficult because her body is more present and takes up more space. She reported struggling with and being anxious about Dance-Movement therapy. According to the somatic experience concept, her mind-body system seemed to be in a state of overactivation (Levine, 1997).

Since she said that relaxing the system by focusing on breathing was not available to her, I offered to experience briefly expanding the lungs through exercises stretching the ribs and thorax – a kind of 'external activation' of the respiratory system that produces expansion and serenity. She arrived at our next meeting with tremors and restlessness, turning her head frequently from side to side. Darry shared the difficulty of leaning back, relaxing, and letting go. She said painfully that she could not remember a time in her childhood when she could rely on someone and feel supported: 'I always had to gather myself up, hold and defend myself against abuse. Or I would run away in my mind and disconnect from my body'.

In relating to the emotion accompanying the possibility of leaning on someone, Darry said that reliance causes her to feel ashamed. She finds it challenging to accept herself as supported or assisted; she does not see a future and does not see herself continuing like that. She added that at that time, her thoughts grew increasingly louder and she could not quiet them using meditation or mindfulness. She experienced dissociations in which she saw herself outside her body: on one hand, she felt relaxed; on the other hand, she injured herself and did not feel pain. She did not think she could go on with the pain involved in her current condition: 'I'd like to completely disconnect from the existence and presence of my body, to nullify like air without feelings, thoughts or emotions'. She added that she calms down at the mere thought of that possibility.

I felt my stomach clenching and concern for her, accompanied by the question of whether she would choose nullification – death. But I also felt a sense of liveliness in her and her presence, a feeling that it is a wish for a silence that can be explored and searched for in the body and stay with it together for a while. I could also hold that concern, knowing that I had partners in keeping her safe and holding her space in the ward. Agreeing to be with her in the nullifying and nothingness later enabled a physical action of grounding, which allowed her to connect to space and time in the present, alongside motoric energy release. She took off her flip-flops so that she could walk barefoot, chose a small physio ball, and began to work with it intensively, dribbling, bouncing, grounding, knee-bending, with creativity, rhythm, and expression. Darry began to share her movement with me, initially without making eye contact; later, she looked at me. When I added music, she kept the rhythm and played with it. In her movement, there was much liveliness; sometimes, she seemed like a little girl enjoying her body, and sometimes like a mature woman dancing in a tribal circle. We both danced, echoing each other's movements and experiencing liveliness and vitality.

Van der Kolk (2015) discussed the collective movement and music that gives a broader context to our lives, noting that universal religious rituals combine rhythmic movements. Levine (1997) described shamanic rituals that use singing and rhythmic dancing to produce an environment where healing occurs. Movement in space and the use of music and rhythms enable the creation of a beat that provides a framework, order, and security and that encourages the mind-body system to move away from stagnation or dissociation. In the Dance-Movement therapy group she participated in, Darry used music to facilitate letting go and having fun; with the music, she felt free to release her overcharged body, feeling grounded by using force and rhythmic treading on the ground. Chaiklin (2016) wrote about the power of the circle that allows, through movement and music, an emotional expression for every individual and a clearer sense of self in the context of a relationship.

Towards her release from the ward, when her anxiety again strengthened, Darry talked about various ways she injured herself until she reached rock bottom and that only then could she start to rise: anorexia, self-inflicted cuts, and occasional sexual relationships with demeaning men who didn't see her. It wasn't until she was trampled entirely that she decided to stop. Again, the desire to die aroused in her a feeling of bliss; she described it as the experience of total control. Again, I felt despair and fear rising in me, but I tried to experience with her the fantasy of complete control over her life and death, holding inside me vitality and hope as well. After remaining in that wish for a while, she said that she wouldn't do it because she wanted to keep living. She raised the idea of removing toxic or repulsive bodily segments, cutting or operating on them, which made me feel reluctant and anxious for her well-being. But before I reacted verbally, she moved on to the desire to dance. Darry could move between the concrete plane of self-injury and the possibility of using movement to symbolically remove toxic parts that had been inserted in her. Upon her release from the ward, she said, 'I've been to a lot of therapy sessions, and I can keep on talking cognitively, but it doesn't seep in. Connecting to my body, with all my fear, enabled a process that was not possible verbally'.

Summary

When victims of sexual trauma arrive at the hospital in extreme states of emotional overwhelm, treatment focuses on stabilising, organisation, regulating, and gaining control. As a casualty of the battle, the body itself initially leads patients to experience various difficulties in meeting and thinking about it. But upon their agreeing to begin listening to it, the body allows them grounding – a connection to reality, a means of identifying impending dissociation and obtaining self-regulation and self-control. The work based on the body's sensory system and the motor system allows a feeling of vitality and presence in the body, releasing the energy stored in the body, exiting the stagnation empowerment, and experiencing a sense of self-efficacy. Combining bodily experiences, anchoring the experiences in language, finding the mediating words, and providing validation within a relationship allows the attainment of control and leaving the psychiatric ward in a slightly more regulated and stable state.

In working with victims of sexual trauma, a therapist must agree to go on a bumpy roller coaster with the patient. To experience with them in the therapist's own body and feelings, the pain and horror, and to hold within the knowledge of hope. To move stagnated parts, flow movement, regulate volume and pain, and repeatedly search for the right way to each one. The Dance-Movement therapy allows the therapists to move with the patients in a spiral movement from stagnation and abuse to the areas of presence and vitality, from the regions of paralysing horror to power and hope. The movement allows for an exit in space, time, and body interchanges.

Note

1 I thank my partners in the focused therapy programme, the psychiatric ward staff for holding space, and Ziv Medical Center's management for supporting the programme.

References

Chaiklin, S. (2016). We dance from the moment our feet touch the earth. In S. Chaiklin & H. Wengrower (Eds.), *The art and science of dance/movement therapy: Life is dance* (pp. 3–12). New York, NY: Brunner Routledge.

Davies, J. M., & Frawley, M. G. (1994). *Treating the adult survivor of childhood sexual abuse: A psychoanalytic perspective.* New York, NY: Basic Books.

Ferenczi, S. (1955). Confusion of tongues between adults and the child. In S. Ferenczi (Ed.), *Final contributions to the problems and methods of psychoanalysis* (pp. 156–167). London: Hogarth Press.

Ferenczi, S. (1995). *The clinical diary.* Cambridge, MA: Harvard University Press.

Fishman, D. (2016). Therapeutic relationships and kinesthetic empathy. In S. Chaiklin & H. Wengrower (Eds.), *The art and science of dance/movement therapy: Life is dance* (pp. 33–54). New York, NY: Brunner Routledge.

Gurevich, H. (2018). The return of dissociation as "absence within absence": Early trauma and dissociation in the tender stage. *Sichot, 32*(2), 134–142 (Hebrew).

Herman, J. L. (1994). *Trauma and recovery: The aftermath of violence—From domestic abuse to political terror.* London: Rivers Oram Press.

Kestenberg-Amighi, J., Loman, S., Lewis, P., & Sossin, K. M. (1999). *The meaning of movement: Developmental and clinical perspectives of the Kestenberg Movement Profile.* New York, NY: Brunner Routledge.

Kleinman, S. (2016). Becoming whole again: Dance/movement therapy for those who suffer from eating disorders. In S. Chaiklin & H. Wengrower (Eds.), *The art and science of dance/movement therapy: Life is dance* (pp. 125–143). New York, NY: Brunner Routledge.

Levine, P. (1997). *Waking the tiger: Healing trauma.* Berkeley, CA: North Atlantic Books.

Lowen, A. (1995). *Joy: The surrender to the body and to life.* London: Penguin Books.

Ogden, T. (1992). *The primitive edge of experience.* New York, NY: Brunner Routledge.

Reich, W. (1972). *Character analysis* (3rd enlarged ed.; V. R. Cartago, Trans.). New York: Farrar, Straus and Giroux (Original work published 1945).

Seligman, T. (2016). Traumatic intersubjectivity, the traumatization of the therapist as an essential process in women and men who were abused in childhood. *Sichot*, *30*(2), 143–150.

Shaham, M. (2017). About movement and non-movement in the therapeutic space with post-traumatic patients. *Beyn-Hamilim*, *12*, 77–96 (Hebrew).

Shahar-Levy, Y. (2004). *From the visible body to the hidden story of the soul: A mind-movement paradigm for dance-movement therapy and the analysis of the language of emotional movement* (2nd ed.). Jerusalem: Self-published (Hebrew).

Shuper Engelhard, E., Pitluk, M., & Elboim-Gabyzon, M. (2021). Reliability and of an observational tool based on grounding quality (Grounding Assessment Tool). *Frontiers in Psychology*, 1–30. https://doi.org/10.3389/fpsyg.2021.621958

Van der Kolk, B. A. (2015). *The body keeps the score: Mind, brain and body in the transformation of trauma*. London: Penguin Books.

Chapter 6

The Dance Not Danced
Working with Movement to Develop Compassionate Relationships and Emotional Growth

Einav Gottlieb-Eliaz

Introduction

This chapter is written from a relational perspective, and using the case study of a young woman, describes both the patient's and the therapist's feelings during movement. It results from the understanding of treatment as a 'joint dance' that evokes transformative physical and psychic feelings in the patient and the therapist which enable a unique, meaningful, and healing therapeutic process to take place.

This chapter will present a movement-based therapeutic process created through work with a young woman, a victim of incest. The thinking about movement in this chapter addresses physical and psychic symptoms, common in therapy with abuse victims: depression, damaged body image, dissociative phenomena, inability to maintain interpersonal relationships, and a sense of grief and loss. Movement interventions described herein attempt to provide a solution to the difficulties characteristic of many victims: difficulty in encountering and sensing their body, difficulty in identifying resources and strengths in their abused body, difficulties in memory and in the ability to maintain a narrative sequence of their lives, difficulty sensing body-mind synchrony with another person without detaching, and difficulty expressing freedom and playfulness in their lives in general, and in relationships, in particular. The interventions I created are a way to experience, using the body's help, and not only words, the pain and the difficulty as well as the attempts at repair and attaining a beneficial bodily experience. The unique combination, between Dance Movement Therapy (DMT) and work with victims of sexual abuse is a natural and obvious combination but at the same time, is also wide-open and complicated. As a dance-movement therapist in this sensitive and complex area, this insight produces and instils within me constant tension. Many victims collect within their bodies unrelenting pain and thus, the body present in the treatment room is experienced as a harsh battlefield. It is therefore natural that treatment of sexual abuse will address the patients' bodily sensations, and will be supported by body-movement work.

DOI: 10.4324/9781003309048-10

The presence of the suffering and wounded body in the therapy room is a significant part of therapy, the ability to talk about the body and to become familiar with its sensations by contemplating its painful, suffering, and disconnected parts enables the victim to explain the body drama in words, to herself and to the therapist; at times it is vague and unclear and at other times, sharp and clear. The fact that the patient can bring and include her scarred body into the therapeutic discourse is, in my view, the beginning of the journey to restoring control over the psychic and physical chaos typical of many victims.

The presence of the body also facilitates the identification of vibrant, strong, and beloved parts in the body of the victim and thus, enables her to find the resources required for the therapeutic journey and the anchors that will assist her in regulating the body during times of distress. It also makes it possible to strengthen the belief that the body is not only a source of suffering and pain but inherently, it possesses the ability to feel sensations of strength, pleasure, and happiness. Van der Kolk (2015) relates to the importance of working with the body and argues that the inability of trauma victims to control what happens in their body, robs them of a basic sense of control. Paralysing bodily symptoms can appear at any given moment, the autonomous nervous system constantly emits false alarms and every encounter with the world can arouse intolerable feelings. The challenge in working with victims is to establish a sense of control over the body and mind and to succeed in coming closer to the areas of trauma without the victim's collapse.

In spite of the advantages of body-movement work in treatment of sexual trauma, the encounter with movement in the room holds the potential for tension and many fears, tension with which I, from my experience as a therapist and supervisor, am familiar. I am of the opinion that the tension is a product of the understanding that the trauma and the movement are opposites with a clear and essential difference; on one side, there is the victim whose life is paved with unceasing attempts to avoid the painful encounter with the debris of trauma. She will do almost anything in order not to encounter a memory, smell, feeling, or body movement which may remind her of the abuse. The life of many victims is a circle of threat from which rescue is not possible, a booby-trapped devil's dance and when the area is mined it is wiser not to move. This feeling of being trapped frequently paralyses victims, makes them constricted, static, and petrified. Many patients enter the therapy room contracted, refuse to remove their coats and place their purse beside them, and at times long months will pass until they are able to relax somewhat in their chair and allow the body release, for even just a moment, from the contraction and gripping. On the other side, there is DMT inviting them on a journey of studying the body, an encounter with familiar and hidden places, trying out new things and wandering in intermediate spaces and less accessible spaces of reality, spaces which may appear to the patient to be unsafe and even dangerous.

In the therapeutic encounter, I often feel that I too am infected by paralysis and restriction and like the patient, I find myself frozen out of fear of hurting, touching, and encountering an intolerable memory and sometimes, even with inaccessible areas in my own psyche. In moments of paralysis, movement is not accessible to me either, any thought or idea concerning working with movement feels imprecise, too vague and sometimes even destabilising and dangerous. More than once, the question of how long must I dwell in the freeze with the patient worked its way into my mind, along with the fear that if we remain here for too much time perhaps we both will freeze to death and will never be able to move again. Seligman (2016) addresses the traumatisation of therapists caring for sexual trauma victims as a fundamental process in therapy. She believes that treating sexual trauma victims becomes possible only when we allow the patient to influence us, to invade and disrupt our status quo. As part of the therapeutic process, the patient must see us, the therapists, succeed in extricating ourselves from being stuck and detached, and from becoming stuck and detached within the relationship, so that she will be able to begin to experience, think, and dream.

Many therapists are concerned with searching for the right and precise moment to emerge from being stuck, to get up from the chair, to give the words a rest and to shift over to movement in the room. I would suggest that it is in fact those moments in which the patient feels the paralysing disconnection in her body, the moments in which the ability to think and react vanish, may be the sign of when to propose movement. These very moments can become an 'act of freedom' (Symington, 1983), an attempt to free oneself from the lasso of the patient's inner world, a destructive lasso which entraps both the therapist and patient. In these moments, I do indeed propose, ask; and, sometimes I feel like a mother of a frightened daughter, holding her patient's hand and saying: 'I know how scary this is, we'll go at your pace, I'm with you, a witness and ally'.

Sarah

Sarah was assaulted in her childhood by a relative and over the years, experienced additional abuse perpetrated by other offenders. When she came to therapy, it was as the result of a deep and lengthy depression which caused her to cease functioning, to get into her bed, to cover herself with a blanket, and disconnect from everything and everyone she loved. I will attempt to describe how, between words, silences, feelings of helplessness, and freezing in the room, I wove in movement which enabled Sarah, for moments at a time, to extricate herself from the detachment and her being stuck, from the feeling of regression and freezing.

The course of therapy

In the initial stages of therapy I frequently used a pouffe, an important accessory in the DMT treatment room. Sarah was lying down on the pouffe and allowing her body to rest, as simple as it is complex, to lay down on a pouffe and try to relax her body. In the background, calm and slow music was playing (always the same melody), and I began to gently touch just the pouffe and to cradle her within it. The initial work centred on the possibility of lying down and afterwards, only to try to intermittingly close her eyes. The ability to lie down on a cradled pouffe, cared for, protected and to try to yield to this experience which, with time, was pleasant and holding for her, was essential to the therapeutic process. It is something we repeatedly returned to and each time Sarah managed to trust me more and more.

The cradling work emerged from a decision to enable regression in the room, to, for a moment, let Sarah retreat into herself within the holding, with very clear boundaries, the pouffe and I delimit the space such that retreat is not infinite and Sarah cannot get lost. The work enabled me to try and create for Sarah a kind of 'primal skin function' (Bick, 1968), a physical-psychic envelope that would unify and hold the parts of her body and mind. Bick, who developed the concept, believed that in mother-infant relations, attuned holding will allow the infant to internalise, with time, the enveloping and containing function and to experience her or his body and mind in an integrative and healthy manner. When, for various reasons, the infant does not receive a good enough primal skin function, the adult is unable to create an integration of all the parts of his or her personality and under the guise of normal functioning, hides a disintegrated personality that cannot live a full life but rather, can only survive in reality.

Also Sarah fell apart after years of relatively good functioning and success in many areas. Outside therapy, she experienced criticism and attacks regarding her mental breakdown, the move away from reality and personal connections. The ability to be in bounded and secure regression in the room, without guilt, was a significant stage in therapy. I hoped that with time Sarah would internalise my holding and be able to on her own produce an integration between the parts of her body and mind, even without the concrete holding in the room.

As work progressed, Sarah continued to lie on the pouffe with her legs close to the wall. Thusly, within the regressive cradling, I asked her to start pushing her legs against the wall while I sat and provided a counterweight on the other side. When she pushed against the wall, I asked her to feel how her body's muscles were beginning to work and to describe to me where in her body she feels strength. With time and patience, the strength would spread to more and more areas in Sarah's body until she succeeded in enlisting her body's strengths and slowly lifting herself to a standing position.

This movement experience accompanied all the initial stages of therapy. Over and over, during several sessions, we returned to the same experience and each time, somewhat different feelings emerged. Sarah wanted to grow and rise to standing on her feet but was afraid and she deliberated. I was not searching for new developments rather, a return to the familiar movement *experiencing* which enabled Sarah to yield to it, to feel safe, and to learn herself through it.

Like many victims, Sarah had problems in the area of memory and the sense of herself. Complete chapters from her childhood disappeared as if they never happened and she felt that she was disconnecting from reality and at times, wandering in worlds of childish imagination and at times, nowhere. This phenomenon, called dissociation, is characteristic of many sexual abuse victims. In dissociation, the victim feels lost, overwhelmed, abandoned, and not connected to the world (Van der Kolk, 2015). The dissociation Sarah experienced caused her to feel unstable, like someone who is not able to feel confident in herself and her emotions, confused and lacking a clear and logical sequence to her life. I suggested to her that using movement, we work on the ability to remember and maintain a sequence of movements. In this intervention, we stood facing each other. Sarah began with her body to produce movement, after which we both repeated her movement. Then I created a movement with my body and we both repeated it. In this way we connected one movement after another, one of Sarah's and one of mine.

In contrast to her feelings in external reality where she does not remember anything and suddenly loses herself, in everything having to do with the movement sequence, Sarah succeeded in feeling present and connected. Already in the first attempts, we succeeded together in creating a long sequence of collaborative movements which we repeated over again with different movement qualities: once slow, once fast, once interrupted, once continuous and flowing, once with music playing, and once with internal music.

Sarah's bodily experience, the ability to maintain a sequence and express it in different ways was moving and brought feelings of life to the room and with it also laughter and playfulness. This work strengthened the closeness and connection between us, a different kind of closeness than the experiencing on the pouffe produced. This time we both stood, together we created a continuous and living dance, a joint creation exclusively Sarah's and mine, in which Sarah's sharpened senses and ability to be present were superb. An invitation to a movement experience which produces a movement sequence, seemingly simple, and yet I would like to suggest that it is challenging and essential for sexual trauma victims in general and for incest victims, in particular. The work on a sequence enables patients to experience the give and take of dialog and listening, relationship qualities which incest victims who endured such difficult developmental trauma never experienced. The playfulness which emerges from the joint work is also valuable for adult victims who were not given the basic right of care-free play. Because children who are abused cease being children something deep within them changes, is vigilant, attunes to the other and matures too soon (Herman, 1992).

The work on the joint sequence allowed Sarah and I to talk about the discrepancy between life outside and life in the therapy room. The feeling that under safe conditions, she maintains the sequence and her memory functions well was very meaningful and with time, Sarah succeeded in tak-ing that safe place with her, out of the room.

Despite the healthy feeling which movement introduced into therapy, Sarah's functioning outside the room was still minimal. Her feelings of guilt were severe and getting in touch with the trauma aroused fear and paralysis. Sarah's life and the therapy, too, were subject to many fluctua-tions and hardships. At that stage I decided to introduce a movement tool into therapy which I had not used before. In my past, I had danced and taught ballroom dancing. I felt that in the sessions with Sarah the emo-tional and physical experience of joint dancing may strengthen her and touch on significant themes with which she was preoccupied. I suggested to Sarah to try out this movement tool out of a wish that our joint harmoni-ous dancing, the attention to small nuances of the body, the ability to trust and be led, will continue to strengthen her, particularly with respect to her ability to establish a place within a relationship.

We started with the rumba, the basic step of the dance is slow and repeti-tive. We practiced it together and alone, again and again, and at the end we produced joint harmonious movement in the room that was based on the ability to stand relatively close to one another and to move in a coordinated way with the utmost attention of one to the movement of the other. The joint dance brought with it a range of emotions. We talked about the diffi-culty of being led and with that, about her yearning to live life with some-one else leading her and taking responsibility for her life and her anguish. Questions concerning dependence, independence and separation, ability to lead, to choose and take responsibility, frustration when the steps become too complicated, and also great sadness and apprehension that she will not be able to attain pleasant and secure harmony in the outside world in which men as well as women hold potential that can lead to abuse and pain.

Therapy ends

Towards the end of therapy, Sarah's ability to express herself in movement became more advanced. In one of the last sessions, when the approach-ing separation was already present in the room, I asked Sarah to move to the 'dance that wasn't danced', everything we did not manage to reach in the therapy and in general, feelings that come up regarding thoughts about having missed out. In their seminal book on therapy with survivors of incest, Davies and Frawley (1994) write that among all adult survivors of childhood sexual abuse, there is a universal phantasy according to which at the moment all the horrific details of the abuse become known, the world will veer off its normal orbit to provide the victim with a new, ideal, and compensatory childhood. One of the harsh insights in therapy with Sarah and in general, was that her childhood will never be repaired and that she must contend with this painful knowledge.

In her book, 'Trauma and Recovery' Herman (2015) also related to the grieving process sexual abuse survivors experience as a fundamental stage in therapy. In her view, mourning is the only way to pay respects worthy of the loss, since there is no fitting compensation. She believed that since the grief is so great, opposing it is a common reason for freezing in advanced stages of therapy. At these points, phantasies may appear regarding a magical solution through revenge, pleas for forgiveness, or compensation. For Sarah, what remained was only the ability to grieve for the harm caused to her, mainly her difficulty to love herself and to love at all.

Sarah danced her feelings of missing out and I sat and was witness to a dance danced in the room that contained so many emotions within it. Sarah moved by herself, freely, in the room, combining different qualities of movement to the sounds of music she chose, and I sat and observed her, witnessing the departing, pained, grieving, angry, and lonely Sarah. But, she was also the Sarah who was coping with her past, discovering herself, daring to dream and desire, more connected to her inner compass, intermittently optimistic, and occasionally happy.

Every now and then I invite a patient to dance the 'dance not danced' which embodies, in different forms, mourning for the childhood taken away and which will not return, but also the ability to move and not freeze, to return to the regions of threat and loneliness though this time, not alone, and to digest the difficult experiences of the past and after many years, to speak of them. I find this movement work very significant. From my perspective, it is therapy come full circle, enabling observation of the therapeutic journey through the body. Many times, in therapy, the beginning of the journey is characterised by the inability to interpret bodily sensations and a difficulty sensing the integration between the body and the mind, while at the end some patients are able to take ownership over their bodily sensations, to connect them to their emotions and to feel the integration necessary for going through this world with a greater sense of security.

At the beginning of this chapter, the discussion revolved around the fundamental contradiction that exists in DMT with victims: the freeze produced by the trauma in contrast with the openness and courage needed in order to feel the body and move in space. I will add that this contrast contains within it a new meaning as well – the patient's ability to move within the therapy and to feel the process in her body enables her to experience, and not only to talk, about the feelings. To experience real cradling and not only to relate to cradling in words and in presence, to experience growth, physically, emerging out of situations of true regressive decline to experience a sequence that exists within and to dance together in harmonious joint movement. All this provides the patient with an additional dimension of comprehension about herself, her pains, her feelings, and her strengths. It likewise enables a significant experience of connection and deep partnership formed in therapy between the patient and the therapist.

Movement creates a new dimension for the therapist as well, a powerful dimension of experiencing the feelings emerging in therapy – the therapist's body is not only a 'symbolic' container, but a real body present, sensitive, and feeling the transitions and implications produced in the room. This sensitive body, which the therapist brings with her into the DMT room enables her to change as a result of the encounter with the patient, to encounter disconnected regions in her own psyche, those she prefers not to touch, to break down, to build back up, to be in pain and become scarred, which makes the work of the therapist unbearable, exhausting, despairing and at the same time, a moving experience and a precious gift.[1]

Note

1 I would like to express my gratitude and appreciation to my supervisor, Yael Lavie, who accompanied me in my therapy of Sarah and who, for me, is a professional inspiration for many years already.

References

Bick, E. (1968). The experience of the skin in early object relations. *The International Journal of Psychoanalysis, 49*, 484–486.

Davies, J. M., & Frawley, M. G. (1994). *Treating the adult survivor of childhood sexual abuse*. New York, NY: Basic Books.

Herman, J. L. (1992). Complex PTSD: A syndrome in survivors of prolonged and repeated trauma. *Journal of traumatic stress, 5*(3), 377–391.

Herman, J. L. (2015). *Trauma and recovery: The aftermath of violence--from domestic abuse to political terror*. Paris: Hachette UK.

Seligman, Z. (2016). Traumatic inter-subjectivity, traumatisation of the therapist as an essential process in treating women and men sexually abused in childhood. *Sichot, 30*(2), 143–150.

Symington, N. (1983). The analyst's act of freedom as agent of therapeutic change. *International Review of Psycho-Analysis, 10*(3), 283–291.

Van der Kolk, B. A. (2015). *The body keeps the score: Brain, mind, and body in the healing of trauma*. London: Penguin Books.

Chapter 7

Identifying and Giving Meaning to Body and Movement Messages in Women Diagnosed with Complex PTSD

Ravit Maltz Schwartz

Introduction

Complex post-traumatic stress disorder (CPTSD) is a psychological disorder which develops in response to an ongoing, repeated experience of interpersonal trauma in a context where the victim cannot escape the abusive situation or stop it. Complex trauma is characterised by three core symptoms: dissociation, somatisation, and emotional regulation difficulties. Dance Movement Therapy (DMT) with patients suffering from CPTSD involves a direct encounter with the body, which represents a 'battlefield'. The body where the trauma occurred carries the traumatic abuse, constantly reminded of it. Often, patients prefer not to relate to the body or not to feel it at all. For some, any thought about the body or even the word 'body', arouses anxiety and re-traumatisation. Using a case study, this chapter describes the way the body and movement undergo transformation, from being the source of the evil to a means of regulation. It illustrates how mirroring, echoing, and validation processes encourage empathy between the therapist and patient and the learning of patterns for safe relations.

This chapter will present the uniqueness of DMT as part of the systematic work conducted in the *LeTsidech* (By Your Side) Department at the *Merhavim* Medical Centre in Israel. This is an inpatient unit for women who have experienced difficult life events and suffer from post-traumatic symptoms expressed, at times, in eating disorder symptoms as well. All of the patients come to the department voluntarily, sleep there but can leave the hospital during the day. The staff includes a range of medical and paramedical professionals working together. Treatment in the department is based on dynamic and psycho-educational models of trauma treatment. The basic assumption is that treatment of trauma cannot be compelled and that restoring control of symptoms to the patient constitutes the key to change. As a safe environment, the department provides a solution to primary needs such as sleep, nutrition, and daily routine alongside needs of belonging and mutual affirmation in a female community.

DOI: 10.4324/9781003309048-11

Therapy is performed in stages, corresponding to Herman's model (2015): the first stage is building a safe space through creating a treatment contract and acquiring tools for coping with the various symptoms. After building a foundation of trust and attaining emotional regulation, the second stage is processing the trauma. The third stage is rehabilitation and return to the community. The department is a therapeutic community with a set of rules designed to protect all of its participants. The patients participate in individual and group therapy which provide a comprehensive solution to intra- and interpersonal emotional difficulties. Referral to groups is adapted to the different therapeutic stages and the patient's preferences: these include dialectical behaviour therapy (DBT), nutrition and body image, dynamic groups, and art therapy groups, among others. In this chapter, using a case study, I will describe how the impairment was expressed in the therapeutic relationship and the nature of work in DMT in situations of complex trauma.

Tamara

Tamara, 35 years of age, was hospitalised in the unit following deterioration in her mental state and dwindling of her functional abilities. A year earlier, she had ceased going to work regularly until finally, she left her work completely. In parallel, she stopped leaving her home, except for the few times she went to medical examinations. Tamara spent the month prior to her hospitalisation in bed. Her waking hours were accompanied by flashbacks and smoking medical marijuana and her sleeping hours were accompanied by nightmares. She ate practically nothing and did not shower.

Tamara is the youngest in a family of three children. Her father was described as a rigid man with a tendency to frequent and unpredictable outbursts. Her mother, a teacher, was described as immersed in her work, practical and demanding. Her parents divorced when she was 16, after a long period of fighting, followed by a period of deafening silence and lack of communication. Her eldest brother was described as the successful child in the family. He succeeded in his studies and in society, and as an adult, he established a family. The middle brother was described as a sociable child who, in his adulthood, settled abroad and did not maintain regular contact with the family.

When she was seven, Tamara was sexually assaulted when her neighbour called to her to come into his home on the pretext of him needing help, and he began to touch her. Tamara told her mother who denied that anything had happened. Tamara's home was not containing and not validating and she preferred to wander around outside, searching for attention, warmth, appreciation, and admiration. During adolescence Tamara was sexually assaulted several more times by different men, some of the abuse continued for some time. As a result, Tamara's functioning was impaired. She mostly wandered the streets and did not go to school. This was how she became acquainted with boys and men, some of whom took advantage of her. These relationships aroused in Tamara a sense of being courted and admired but also led to a decrease in her feelings of self-worth and an increase in self-destructive behaviours.

With time, symptoms of night terrors, hyper-vigilance, and self-harm increased. At age 12, a series of disorders began such as body dysmorphia, a marked reduction in eating, a drastic reduction in weight, and anxiety concerning a return to normal weight. Her parents did not notice but one of her teachers helped refer her to treatment where she was diagnosed as suffering from restrictive anorexia nervosa, a type of eating disorder. Treatment led to an improvement in the symptoms of the eating disorder, though the fluctuations between reduction and expansion continued in other areas of life.

About a year before the hospitalisation, Tamara experienced a sexual assault perpetrated by a friend of her father. As a young girl, Tamara had known him and was therefore happy to greet him at a social event. He complimented her on her appearance and suggested they meet again. Tamara, who was pleased by his interest in her, was happy to set another meeting with him. These moments in which Tamara received attention and interest blocked her judgement and left her without the ability to think about the impropriety of a date with him. He collected her from her home on the way to some entertainment, the travel to which on side roads explained away as a way of showing her a beautiful observation point. When they arrived there he began to touch her. As for the rest of the incident, Tamara does not remember. She disconnected, and later found herself injured and bleeding at the entrance to her home.

Tamara did not tell her family about the assault. Unconsciously, she blamed her father for the attack and began to be aggressive and violent towards him. The father severed relations with her after she lodged a complaint against him with the police for violence. Her eldest brother was angry about her behaviour towards the father and he too severed ties with her. Her mother arrived to care for her only when Tamara actively expressed suicidal thoughts, but when she was hospitalised she avoided contact with her. Tamara tended to extreme shifts from moments where she blamed the environment for her situation to moments in which she felt she was to blame for every possible thing. Self-harm served to calm her and as a way to punish herself and those around her. In this way, she 'forced' her family to relate to her and take care of her. During the hospitalisation Tamara was diagnosed as suffering from complex post-trauma, borderline personality disorder, and from a non-specific eating disorder.

The course of therapy

At the first session, Tamara entered the treatment room with suspicion, her gaze surveyed the room and she sat down on the easy chair. She immediately crossed her legs so that her top leg rested on the lower one, in a way that closed the space between the armrests of the easy chair. I wondered about the type of sitting and its implicit message. She may be saying that she is not ready to meet me or perhaps she is saying that she is afraid of the encounter, or possibly she is defining the personal space she needs. Tamara found it difficult to tell about herself, something that was in line with the closed space she created by the position of her body. In practice, she spoke of general things. She complained about the conditions in the unit and the lack of the staff's attention, that they do not see her, about her difficulties and the complexity of what she contends with. As she spoke her complaints, she looked directly at me with menacing eyes.

The many complaints and the look in her eyes aroused in me a sense of attack and a need to be protected and safeguarded. This was a 'taste' of the expectations Tamara had of those surrounding her and a message to me with respect to the difficulty of making a connection. Tamara needed precise attunement to her and a gradual building of the relationship in order to let go and come closer. Since we were just at the beginning of our relationship, I chose not to reflect these understandings but I validated her difficult experience. Giving validation caused her to feel more understood and promoted a safe therapeutic relationship – the first stage in Herman's (2015) therapeutic process.

My validation of her anger provided Tamara with a safe environment to express herself. Giving an explanation for her complaints, in that this was the beginning of therapy which requires a space for become acquainted and adjustment to life in the unit – a new framework, part of which was relinquishing personal space that she was accustomed to and acceptance of the unit's rules (such as attending meals, functioning in groups, sleep at night and not during the day, life with a large group of patients), provided an explanation her the difficulty she experienced. Consideration of the difficulties in the unit aroused in Tamara feelings and memories of deprivation and injustice in her life. She remembered a situation in which her parents hosted friends and her father called for her eldest brother and was proud of his capabilities, his success in studies and society and even remarked on his beauty. The memory aroused great pain and anger concerning her parents' inability to see her many efforts to feel wanted within the family. It provoked an experience of feeling ugly and that she would never be able of attracting her parents' gaze. In similar moments in which she felt frustration, invisibility, and lack of attention, such as she felt when she entered the unit, immediately brought up the same familiar emotions of lack of respect and self-worth. Those same harsh emotions represented a ground for other unsatisfying interpersonal experiences in which she learned to place herself in the position of the victim. This position is related to the emotional system produced in pathological identifications within a complex internalisation system, and serves as a survival mechanism, developed in the face of trauma (Davies & Frawley, 1994). According to Davies and

Frawley, many survivors of complex trauma hold a characteristic structure of defences which includes splitting, denial, acting out, omnipotence, projective identification, and dissociation.

In the therapeutic process a kind of ritual was created wherein at the beginning of each session, Tamara sat with her legs crossed. The more established our relationship became, the more Tamara could engage in greater direct eye contact with me for longer periods and the more she could see in my gaze that I see her, the crossing of her legs became more relaxed. Her sitting position changed, became somewhat freer and less closed within the easy chair. That is, the relationship became a little more flexible, Tamara began to feel more confident in my presence and relied on my eyes to accompany her and on my voice as a voice which accompanies the process she was going through in therapy. At this stage, her body space remained rather limited and did not allow spontaneous movement. The absence of spontaneous movement is instructive regarding unprocessed emotional trauma related to an experience of bodily freeze.

Tamara's physical reactions when faced with situations of pain and frustration were characterised by constriction, drawing her shoulders in towards her chest, lowering her head, and repetitive movement of her upper leg. Since the body in the easy chair was also a 'talking body', I turned her attention to what takes place in her body when expressing frustration, pain, and injustice. Turning her focus to her body triggered great pain for her. Her entire body hurt and grieved in the face of her attempts to connect. The body's attention was swept directly into trauma and aroused in her, immediately, traumatic memories and a catastrophic fall to re-enactment of the trauma (Davies, 2004).

Looking back on the development of the therapeutic relationship, it can be seen that when I suggested that attention be turned to the body, it led Tamara to experience intolerable pain. This suggestion put me in the position of the attacker, rousing in me, as the therapist, great fear, guilt, and a sense of helplessness. Darwin (1872) first related to the relationship between the body and the mind and claimed that the emotions are the source driving action and they are expressed, mainly, in facial and body muscles. In practice, the goal of the feelings is to cause muscular movement which will restore the organism to a situation of safety and balance. Van der Kolk (2014) found that there are reciprocal relations between the heart, intestines, and brain via the vagal nerve which connects many organs, including: the brain, lungs, heart, stomach, and intestines. Trauma survivors focus muscle energy on the attempt to suppress the inner chaos and strong emotions from which they suffer, at the expense of spontaneous involvement in their lives. This leads to an understanding of trauma survivors' great desire to numb their senses and feelings, which, over time, leads to bodily pain (Porges, 2001).

Merleau-Ponty, who studied the place of the body in philosophy relates to the living body as the subject's point of origin with respect to the world and from which every interaction is determined, whether the subject vis-a-vis him or herself, or with respect to the environment (Iwakuma, 2002). He argues that unlike other objects in the world, the body is always involved in the surrounding world and therefore the body is experiential. According to him, the subject does not passively perceive the world but rather with his or her body, creates the movement in the time and space expanses.

In stark contrast to a healthy state, people who have experienced ongoing trauma have learnt to 'shut off' regions of the brain responsible for transmitting emotional and sensory information, which leads to disruption in sensory recording. As a result, the structures responsible for identifying experiences of the self and self-identification may become impaired (Bluhm et al., 2009). Without recording sensations, the formulation of experiences of the self is compromised. Hence, when the self-sensing system breaks down, ways must be found to restore it so that it functions, in order for the individual to be able to know where he is and to be conscious of what is happening to him. Only in this way will he be able to feel his self as present (Van der Kolk, 2014). The body is the key to treatment and healing of trauma, and without in-depth exploration of bodily expression, comprehension of the field of trauma remains limited (Leavitt, 2008; Ogden, Minton, & Pain, 2006).

Ogden (2001) explains that in analysis, healthy development is tied to the patient's ability to be alive in his body. He stresses that achieving a sense of mind-body integration is more problematic for people who, in early childhood, suffered from neglect or trauma. This difficulty stems from an attempt to manufacture control by abolishing dependence on another, self-blame and a sense of omnipotence. Using Bick's (1968) definition, this can be seen as creating a 'second skin', a defensive configuration in which the dependence on the object is replaced by pseudo-independence. This is a pathological and omnipotent pattern whose aim is to control every layer of bodily and interpersonal experience and to nullify experiences which are not controlled. In light of the fact that interpersonal relations become records in the body, treatment of trauma victims must relate to the bodily dimension.

DMT with victims of complex trauma arouses much difficulty with patients. Herman (2015) explains that (female) trauma victims feel unsure within their own bodies to the point where it seems to them that their emotions and thoughts are out of control. They also feel unsure with respect to others. Gur (2015) adds that due to the trauma which was, inherently, a breaking of boundaries, victims have difficulty maintaining boundaries of the self and the boundaries of their bodies. In light of their experience of a violated and insecure body, many times trauma victims tend to deny the body and its existence, as an attempt to set boundaries that were breached.

This was also the case with Tamara, where every attention to the body aroused, immediately, physical pain. In these moments, her body appeared like a single block operating inclusively, with no ability to separate organs and to distinguish between sensations. The pain caused her body's muscles to contract and appear even more vigilant and rigid. Her breathing rate increased and with every inhale less and less air was consumed and her gaze became flat. For Tamara, turning attention to her body provoked intolerable sensations and a re-enactment of the trauma was created, with her being swallowed within it. There was no body to which to relate, what remained was only the disconnection and an amorphous, dissociative experience appeared.

The dissociative mechanism expresses a spectrum of states from distancing to disconnection which protects against feelings, sensations, experiences, and memories emanating from the flow of consciousness and memory (Bernstein, Putnam, Espírito-Santo, & Pio-Abreu, 1986). Due to the dissociation, the overwhelming experience is split to shards of sounds, feelings, visions, thoughts, and sensations which invade the present and are repeatedly replayed (Van der Kolk, 2014). The experience of threat is experienced as something that can return at any moment with no knowledge of when it will occur and with no ability to defend against it. The threat is, first and foremost, bodily, and owing to this, the emphasis in therapeutic work is on creating a space for gradual work with the body. In therapy with Tamara, the re-enactment of the trauma occurred as a result of turning the attention to the body, provoking an undifferentiated pain, following which she and I both felt as if we were on a slippery wall with no place to grab onto, as we fall into an shadowy abyss, a 'nameless dread', in the language of Bion (2018). The term serves Bion in describing an extreme measure of threat in early childhood, created when the figure caring for the infant is incapable of containing his projection. The infant senses a threat which does not acquire meaning and therefore, he internalises a nameless dread instead of processing the fear in a way that makes it tolerable. As mentioned, in these moments, Tamara's body became rigid, immobile, her shoulders were drawn towards her chest, her head was lowered and her eyes shut or their gaze was averted and became flat. Her breathing was more rapid and more frequent and her leg continued to move restlessly. Neither one of us understood the meaning of the threat yet. Tamara was sucked into the trauma as a victim while I was introduced into it as the aggressor. Each one in her place felt psychic pain, detachment, panic, and fear.

When a person encounters something that reminds her of a threatening situation, as happened to Tamara when I drew her attention to her body, all of the body's emergency systems (sympathetic nervous system) begin to act. More primitive regions of the brain take charge and developed regions, such as the cortex, responsible for rational thought and processing, are less involved. As a result, the person is less aware of the situation in which she finds herself but her body becomes active in planning to flee or to fight, and at times, to freeze, which are pre-programmed in the primitive regions of the brain. To the extent that the escape plan succeeded and the danger was forgotten, the body can return to its inner balance which allows bodily presence in the present. In cases where the natural flight response is blocked, like in Tamara's assault, the brain continues to send messages to the body that it is still in a threatened state (Lima et al., 2010). In this case, the body entered a freeze state and only Tamara's leg continued to move as if it were searching for an escape route, constituting a discharge of energy (Levine, 1997).

As this was a patient who had experienced complex traumatic events, her emergency system was very sensitive to reactivation, and any minor stimulus could arouse powerful and unregulated reactions. Moreover, since the meaning of the threat provoked had not yet been clarified in the therapeutic process there was a need to go back and anchor Tamara's experience in the present and restore control to her. I therefore attempted to create grounding using a connection to the 'here and now'. Grounding in DMT relates to the nature of the psycho-physical presence in the 'here and now' and to the experience of physical and emotional support the person feels in the world (Guest, Parker, & Williams, 2019; Hilton, 2012).

For Tamara, the connection to the body aroused restlessness and as such, I tried using grounding through the senses. At first I asked her to acknowledge that she was hearing me. She nodded her head. I then asked her to place her hands on the cold, metallic armrests of the easy chair and I drew her attention to the coldness. At the same time, I reminded her where we were, encouraged her to move her toes and fingers in order to introduce controlled movement and afterwards, I asked her to check whether she could open her eyes just a slit's-worth. When her eyes opened a little I suggested to her to move her head a little so that she can peruse the room with her eyes. In this way, I emphasised the sensory experience taking place in the here and now.

In his article on the 'autistic-contiguous position', Ogden (2018) explains that sensory experience is at the core of the ability to attribute meaning to experience. He adds that sensory experience on the skin's surface has a decisive influence on the infant's development since it represents the site on which the pre-symbolic world coalesces, which is principally comprised of sensory imprints (the unique shape created in the individual when her skin encounters another thing) with the interpersonal world. In practice, I tried to help Tamara pay attention to the sensory imprint she creates in the meeting of her hand with the metal arms of the chair and in doing so, to create a 'felt shape', as Tustin (2018) defines it. A felt shape is the impression and the recording which the body's sensation creates. This is not the actual shape of the object but a shape we sense it to be. This was the manner in which we halted the tailspin into the trauma and began to construct a new space in which it was possible to investigate the dissociative process. By means of this investigation, Tamara was able to break the tailspin, observe feelings and sensations that were aroused within her and to try and understand the context in which they were produced. Thus began processing of the trauma, the second stage in Herman's (2015) therapeutic process.

The interpersonal interaction between Tamara and myself formed a basis for creation of a sensory surface. The sensory surface connecting Tamara and myself conferred on her feelings of safety, trust, and a certain control. That is to say, therapy represented a space in which Tamara activated her body's sensory system in the aim of paying attention to her presence in the body at a specific moment and by relying on the relationship between us. Through this, sensory surfaces were built which formed anchors of security and regulation in our relations, and which established the work on processing the trauma without being dragged into it. The more these experiences continued to be built and the therapeutic space became more secure, moderate, and regulated, remembering of traumatic situations was facilitated, which also involved more developed regions of the brain that allow observation of the experience.

Tamara's sense of security in me and in the unit grew and was expressed by her willingness to begin to open up the trauma while controlling the dosage of 'contact' with the trauma. In parallel, she decided to move from the familiar armchair. She relocated to sitting on the carpet with her back leaning on the pouffe. It appeared that she needed stable ground and soft and enveloping support. This positioning can be identified as compatible with the 'parental-envelope setting', a concept coined by Shahar-Levy (2009), which refers to a wrapped and embraced body in need of external moorings. In parallel, I too moved my position to the carpet but without a backrest. I chose to sit at an angle of about 75 degrees from her, in the aim of creating a partial 'facing-ness' which is not direct. Unlike the parental-envelope setting, the 'face-to-face setting' envelope relates to the body's ability to support itself from within and to be separate from the other in relations. Face-to-face symbolises the separation in experience and perception (Shahar-Levy). My positioning was conscious, in order to create eye contact, at the same height as Tamara, and to encourage reciprocity and at the same time, to be a role model as well – with respect to the body's ability to support itself.

This period was accompanied by dreams and flashbacks from the different assaults she went through and particularly from the assault that occurred the preceding year. In therapy, Tamara managed to talk about parts of dreams she dreamt and in general, was more successful in regulating herself and not being completely swept up in the trauma. By sharing her experiences she was not left alone, as happened during her traumatic assaults. This sharing enabled delving deeper into the different experiences and building the context and narrative of the events of her life.

An important part of the process was based on validating the various feelings that arose, while also developing the ability to bear, distinguish, name, and articulate them.

Tamara shared the sense of foreboding she had before she went out with her father's friend. The sharing aroused great anger with herself for going with him despite her feelings. She was angry about having gotten into that situation, about not understanding that going out with a person so much older than herself was inviting danger, about not fleeing from there or fighting him, and about allowing the inappropriate contact when she said only in a weak voice that she wants him to stop but did not do anything besides that. These memories led her to conclude that she caused the various men to rape her and that she is to blame for everything that happened to her. In her understanding, she was assaulted without any resistance on her part.

These memories, contemplations, and feelings brought up past traumas and we could, together, examine her childhood and adolescence. She understood that she wanted to be accepted, to get close to certain boys so that they would value her and love her. We discovered that, as a child, she yearned for someone to see her, understand her, to relate to her, and value her. By enlarging the area of focus, her unfulfilled needs as a young girl appeared. At this stage of the therapy, Tamara allowed me to walk with her on the paths of her childhood and thus, together, we could understand her pain as a girl and produce an explanation and interpret why she found herself in this abusive situation.

Understanding her behaviour as a girl functioning in an unprotected world with needs for love and closeness which were not sufficiently met, brought us to address her relationships with members of her nuclear family. We had identified that since childhood she felt jealous of her eldest brother, we understood that at home she did not receive the warmth, containment, and love she needed and that her parents spent many hours at work and she was left on her own. We discovered that the main way she received attention from her parents was through illness. Tamara's core pattern for generating closeness was through the 'role of the patient' and she did not find other ways to express herself other than in this role. Anger surfaced, great helplessness and censoriousness regarding the ways to which she was compelled to resort in order bring others closer. She blamed everyone in that they brought her to this state. She again reached the sweeping conclusion that the other is never benevolent. In parallel, when the question lodged itself between us, she expressed anxiety concerning the closeness created between us, whether I too would abandon her, as happened in her past relationships.

These fears made their presence felt in the room, leading her to become increasingly passive. During this period, she leaned more and more on the pouffe behind her. She interpreted my every movement as my desire to distance myself from her and thus my desire not to be with her any longer. I felt trapped by her fears and that I could not move. I would sit, immobile, until my legs became numb, out of unconscious knowledge that every movement was dangerous. Our relations, too, entered a state of stagnation, non-movement. On the one hand, a safe and static space was created, and on the other, I felt that this space was closing in on us. I felt as if I were trapped in a loop of guilt and blame. I was caught in Tamara's covert 'lasso'. Symington (1983) explains that the patient uses a covert lasso, enabling her to gain control over the therapist and bind him far from the arena of acknowledgement of the trauma and its processing. The therapist feels blocked and deprived of the freedom to spontaneously move. This lasso represented the image of the relations Tamara knew how to create in her relations, and my body served as the means of input for the sensations and sensory messages uncovered in the relational space between myself and Tamara.

The change occurred after I became conscious of the sense of entrapment and I gathered courage to try and extricate myself from it. I began to introduce miniscule changes into our shared space, such as a change in my sitting position and slight movement of my legs, small degrees of moving closer or further from Tamara. The mental release enabled me to also somewhat free my body and movement and to change my position in our shared sitting space. Symington describes this as an 'act of freedom' which, for the therapist, brings about inner mental freedom.

These changes aroused aggressiveness and withdrawal on Tamara's part, while blame was placed on me. She said to me: 'I don't interest you anymore', 'You want to get rid of me'. Despite the anger towards me, I encouraged Tamara to express her feelings regarding the changes created in our shared space. Tamara expressed anger, humiliation, and fear of abandonment. These feelings were familiar to us both, but for the first time we were able to touch on the phantasy of permanent relations that do not change, which can change only when she wishes it, while the other must adapt himself to her, completely.

Tamara seemed to try and turn the other into a sensory surface that would contain her in a totally safe and attuned manner. Her demand was for a constant sensory surface where no other has space to change it at all. In her past, her self-harm constituted the constant and safe sensory surface which was not dependent on any other person and even provided secondary gain, in that it drew attention away from the harm that occurred in relationships. The ability to bear her aggression without panicking and even accepting it while giving meaning to fear, frustration, desire to be seen, and thought, helped create a broadening of our relationship and a beginning of flexibility. All this represented a possibility for building a new space to investigate the distances in the therapeutic relationship. Movement began to be an actual option.

First, there was a need to get up off the carpet. For this, I used a ceremony we had fashioned at the end of each therapy session in order to rise prior to leaving the room. To do so there was a need for a transition from the closed space of our relations, in the sitting position, to a surface of standing on our feet. This transition required Tamara to shift from the 'enveloped' sitting to a vertical state of 'facing-ness', which possesses self-containment. The transition from the ground to elevation is a transition which necessitates support. In order to emphasise this transition, I suggested trying to get up by extending our hands to one another and getting up while our hands are connected and supporting the other. Mutual support prevents appeal to object-based support (inanimate objects). In this manner, the difficulty, the coping, and the transition from a sitting state to a standing state remain within the relationship. Since we were both in need of support, it required a mutual rising where success or non-success was joint. And indeed, we found it difficult to be synchronised. At times, Tamara did not manage to get up, and at times, it was I who could not. It took some time until we found our own rhythm for rising which included a degree of reliance on the self and a degree of reliance on the other. This synchrony was part of a shared secure rhythm where listening to the inside and outside took place in the attempt to create a mutual relationship. The experience emphasised the self-containment ability within relations with the other, something which was not possible in the past, where breakdown and collapse occurred following a yearning for the other to attune himself to and contain her.

From this position, we began to move around the room and examine options for closeness and distance. At first, only I went around and she stood in place. In moving, I was exposed to Tamara's wish that I'd know precisely when I need to come a little closer to her without her expressing her will in words. Many times I missed it and did not know I was to come closer. In these cases, her disappointment was expressed in rage. Our shared and ongoing relationship made it possible to abide the frustration in the room and to continue trying.

Through these attempts, the immense pain and complex impairment in early relations Tamara bore could be understood. We had a better understanding of the helplessness she experienced and experiences in moments when she is not understood, and in this way we were able to get in touch with her wish that her needs be precisely known without having to express them. We discovered that the pattern of using her 'sick' body was a tool for creating connections because it had never allowed development of the ability to settle into a spontaneous and vital body.

This being the case, I suggested to Tamara that she try, in therapy, to express her needs in real time. Tamara felt fear, together with a willingness to try. Expression of a desire for closeness aroused feelings of threat and paralysis in Tamara. She understood that her method of bringing people close to her was through creating a provocative incident: suicide attempts, self-harm, pains, and addictions, and that the way to create such incidents was through using her body as tool. Tamara did not feel as though she had the option of creating closeness in any other way. Recognition of these needs in the protected therapeutic space led to other attempts at closeness. In the beginning, she did not succeed in moving from her place. Just the thought of a slight move closer to me in the space, while I do not move closer to her, aroused danger and fear of rejection. Physical closeness brought up the wish for a relationship and exposed her to the vulnerability which exists in relationships.

For her, the question arose: Why give up her methods for creating closeness, and alongside this, an existential anxiety arose of fear of abandonment and threatening and terrifying loneliness. She understood that if she relinquished her self-harm she would be demonstrating to those around her that she was mature enough to manage on her own and as such, she would still be left alone and desolate. In parallel, the disadvantages of self-harm also surfaced, while relating to the personal and interpersonal costs she paid for it. She understood that those close to her already tended to avoid closeness to her in the ways she invited it, and a new and intense pain arose owing to the fear of the lack of knowledge concerning how to create and maintain relations with others.

These understandings brought about a tempering of our shared sensory surface and changed the rhythm which had characterised our relationship. Tamara agreed to a situation in which we both move, one towards the other or move away from one another. In this way, we created attuned rhythmic movement in which we were both active. In Tustin's (2018) terms, this can be defined as a 'safe rhythm', a new rhythm which develops from the diverse mother and infant rhythms, from sensory, physical and emotional interaction which becomes a wellspring of shared creation for them both. Porges (2001) explains that the autonomous nervous system is comprised of three regulatory systems: the social engagement system, the sympathetic nervous system, and the parasympathetic nervous system. The level of a person's sense of security in any given moment determines which of the systems will operate. When a person feels threatened he first turns to the social engagement system where he will try to attain a sense of security by asking for help and support from people around him. In the event the individual does not attain the desired assistance or in situations of immediate danger, the sympathetic nervous system will be activated to engage in fight or flight actions. In the event that there is no possibility for flight or fight, the person is trapped or forcibly held, operation of the parasympathetic system is initiated to achieve a state of freeze or faint (collapse).

According to this theory, the social engagement system developed in mammals in order to support social life and is the basis of survival. In practice, in order to experience emotional closeness to others, the person must temporarily inactivate his defence systems. For Tamara, it was too dangerous to inactivate her defence system and as such the possibility of emotional closeness was lacking. In light of the therapeutic relationship where relations of trust and security were established, we were able to try out movements of coming closer. During the course of the attempts I was attuned to her rhythm of movement and to her: to the distance of the body's organs from one another, to the flow of movement, to muscle tension and generally, to the way Tamara's body was held. In parallel, I organised the experience in the room using a soft voice and with phrases accompanying the experience.

The joint movement activated the social engagement system and created a rhythm of security based on kinaesthetic empathy. That is to say, a joint activity that created an opening to experience the other's inner life (Fischman, 2015). Neurologists have found that empathy is a physiological phenomenon (Iacoboni, 2009). That is, the ability to understand others is biologically embedded as a primal form of mirroring based on the primal connection between the parent and infant. Mirror neurons provide the basis for the ability to understand something about the experience of the other without having to actually perform the same action. This is the basis of empathic ability (Meltzoff & Prinz, 2002).

DMT has significant clinical influence on the psychotherapeutic implications of mirror neuron activity (Berrol, 2006). Research has found an increase in the activity of mirror neuron circuits following learning a dance (Calvo-Merino, Glaser, Grèzes, Passingham, & Haggard, 2004). During the course of DMT there is use of mirroring, echoing, and imitation of movement while attending to the degree of muscle tension, flow of movement, body posture, range of movement, and additional parameters which express layers of the patient's personal story. All these engage the mirror neurons and increase the empathic ability and the ability to understand the other (Fischman, 2015). Similarly, the movement experiences Tamara and I engaged in enabled microscopic listening to the body's sensations, which were the beginning of settling in the body and identifying self and mutual bodily signals. The structural process of the movement brought about an attempt and a formation of a more benevolent relationship and promoted thinking about leaving the unit. The rehabilitation stage which is the last stage in therapy, according to Herman (2015), did not take place in the classic sense, as a stage unto itself, but the intentions to rehabilitate as well as preparation for continuing the process outside the unit were taking place all the time, in parallel to processing the trauma.

In summary, in this case description, the difficulties involved in work with victims of complex trauma, in general and work using DMT, in particular, can be seen. Attendance to the body, to sensory messages, and to feelings is a complicated task. A slow process, observational, accepting and validating, leads to the beginning of control and emotional regulation. These regulation processes are the basis for getting in touch with complex feelings of guilt and shame, inherent elements of traumatic abuse. The interpersonal experience in the therapy room, which includes study of emotional and physical processes allows an integrative and inclusive reading of the trauma and its various recordings. This joint process leads to construction of a personal narrative of life events, comprehension and even a start to accepting difficult life events.

Movement experiences constitute a real change engine for interpersonal relations and for a transition from a traumatic body to a body that can bear itself and sometimes even listen to 'news flashes' that surface and emerge from it and tell something of the experience taking place at that very moment. DMT summons experiencing in an interpersonal encounter and in a spontaneous movement experience in the therapy room. The emphasis is on movement, bodily and empathic listening which constitutes another, benevolent and real relationship. DMT with survivors of complex trauma confronts the patient with her body, from which many of them wish to be 'released'. The traumatic body, aching, stresses the physical and psychic pains which brought about the development of mechanisms of reduction, halting, fear of movement, rigidity, and fixation. It is a powerful encounter, at times too direct and at times too painful, but critical for the healing process and the attainment of security and control.[1]

Note

1 I would like to thank Dr. Inbal Shlomi, director of the '*LeTsidech*' Department at the *Merhavim* (formerly Be'er Yaacov) Medical Centre, to Kay Birenbaun Itsikson, clinical psychologist and instructor, the LeTsidech Department at the Merhavim Medical Centre, and to Keren Sagiv, clinical dietician, LeTsidech Department at the Merhavim Medical Centre.

References

Bernstein, E. M., Putnam, F. W., Espírito-Santo, H., & Pio-Abreu, J. L. (1986). Dissociative experiences scale. *Dissociation*, 6, 16–23.

Berrol, C. (2006). Neuroscience meets dance/movement therapy: Mirror neurons, the therapeutic process and empathy. *The Arts in Psychotherapy*, 33(4), 302–315.

Bick, E. (1968/1988). The experience of the skin in early object-relations. In E. BottSpillius (Ed.), *Melanie Klein today, volume 1: Mainly theory – Developments in theory and practice* (pp. 187–191). New York, NY: Brunner Routledge.

Bion, W. R. (2018). A theory of thinking. In W. R. Bion (Ed.), *Second thoughts: Selected papers on psycho-analysis*. New York, NY: Brunner Routledge.

Bluhm, R. L., Williamson, P. C., Osuch, E. A., Frewen, P. A., Stevens, T. K., Boksman, K., ... Lanius, R. A. (2009). Alterations in default network connectivity in post-traumatic stress disorder related to early-life trauma. *Journal of Psychiatry & Neuroscience*, 34(3), 187.

Calvo-Merino, B., Glaser, D. E., Grèzes, J., Passingham, R. E., & Haggard, P. (2004). Action observation and acquired motor skills: An FMRI study with expert dancers. *Cerebral Cortex*, 15(8), 1243–1249.

Darwin, C. (1872). *Der Ausdruck der Gemüthsbewegung bei dem Menschen und den Thieren*. E. Schweizer.

Davies, J. M. (2004). Whose bad objects are we anyway? Repetition and our elusive love affair with evil. *Psychoanalytic Dialogues*, 14(6), 711–732.

Davies, J. M., & Frawley, M. G. (1994). *Treating the adult survivor of childhood sexual abuse*. New York, NY: Basic Books.

Fischman, D. (2015). Therapeutic relationships and kinesthetic empathy. In S. Chaiklin, & H. Wengrower (Eds.), *The art and science of dance/movement therapy: Life is dance*. Routledge. *The art and science of dance/movement therapy* (pp. 65–84). New York, NY: Routledge.

Guest, D., Parker, J., & Williams, S. L. (2019). Development of modern bioenergetic analysis. *Movement and Dance in Psychotherapy*, *14*(4), 264–276.

Herman, J. L. (1992). Complex PTSD: A syndrome in survivors of prolonged and repeated trauma. *Journal of Traumatic Stress*, *5*(3), 377–391.

Herman, J. L. (2015). *Trauma and recovery: The aftermath of violence – From domestic abuse to political terror*. Hachette UK, Basic Books.

Hilton, R. (2012). The ever changing constancy of body psychotherapy. *International Body Psychotherapy Journal*, *11*(2), 74–93.

Iacoboni, M. (2009). *Mirroring people: The new science of how we connect with others*. Farrar: Straus and Giroux.

Iwakuma, M. (2002). The body as embodiment: An investigation of the body by Merleau-Ponty. *Disability, Postmodernity, Embodying Disability Theory*, *1*, 76–87.

Leavitt, K.S. (2008). Pat Ogden, Kekuni Minton and Clare Pain, Trauma and the body: A sensorimotor approach to psychotherapy. *Clinical Social Work Journal*, *36*, 221–223. https://doi.org/10.1007/s10615-007-0141-1

Levine, P. A. (1997). *Waking the tiger: Healing trauma: The innate capacity to transform overwhelming experiences*. Berkeley, CA: North Atlantic Books.

Lima, A. A. Fiszman, A., Marques-Portella, C., Mendlowicz, M. V., Coutinho, E. S., Maia, D. C., ... Figueira, I. (2010). The impact of tonic immobility reaction on the prognosis of posttraumatic stress disorder. *Journal of Psychiatric Research*, *44*(4), 224–228.

Meltzoff, A. N., & Prinz, W. (Eds.). (2002). *The imitative mind: Development, evolution and brain bases* (Vol. 6). Cambridge: Cambridge University Press.

Ogden, P., Minton, K., & Pain, C. (2006). *Trauma and the body: A sensorimotor approach to psychotherapy (Norton series on interpersonal neurobiology)*. New York: WW Norton & Company.

Ogden, T. H. (2001). Re-minding the body. *American Journal of Psychotherapy*, *55*(1), 92–104.

Ogden, T. H. (2018). *The autistic-contiguous position. The primitive edge of experience*. New York, NY: Routledge.

Porges, S. W. (2001). The polyvagal theory: Phylogenetic substrates of a social nervous system. *International Journal of Psychophysiology*, *42*(2), 123–146.

Shahar-Levy, Y. (2009). Emotorics: A psychomotor model for the analysis and interpretation of emotive motor behavior. In S. Chaiklin & H. Wengrower (Eds.), *The art and science of dance/movement therapy* (pp. 275–307). New York, NY: Routledge.

Symington, N. (1983). The analyst's act of freedom as agent of therapeutic change. *International Review of Psycho-Analysis*, *10*(3), 283–291.

Tustin, F. (2018). The rhythm of safety 1. In F. Tustin (Ed.), *Autism in childhood and autistic features in adults* (pp. 187–202). New York, NY: Routledge.

Van der Kolk, B. (2014). *The body keeps the score: Mind, brain and body in the transformation of trauma*. London: Penguin.

Chapter 8

Intergenerational Transmission of Sexual Abuse from Mother to Son

Orit Etzion-Rosenberg

Introduction

This chapter describes attributes of non-verbal communication involved in intergenerational relations. Content that did not receive place and words in the patient's life manifested in the therapy room, and through bodily experiences told the story of the primal dyad. A case description illustrates how, by attending to the body and to non-verbal communication, words can be given to primal experiences stemming from the trauma.

Through the bodily experience in counter-transference, place and words can be given to primal experiences which emanate from trauma. By paying attention to the body and non-verbal communication conveyed through it, it is possible to observe transference processes and the emotional and physical 'memory clusters' (Shahar-Levy, 2004) stored in the patient's body. In the case description presented in this chapter, the cluster is related to disgust and invasiveness.

In her book, *These Parents Who Live Through Me*, Gampel (2010) describes the psychological influences of the Holocaust using a metaphor of radioactive matter: matter without form, odour, or colour, which invades but cannot be directly perceived, yet its effects are not limited in time and space. Exposure to radiation can cause diverse and unexpected manifestations in the body. This could also describe the impact of ongoing sexual trauma in childhood. Childhood trauma impacts the personality formation of an abused child who, later, as a mother, communicates with her son through these 'radioactive' materials, to which she has no access and are conveyed without words in the primal dyad. Yarom (2010), in her book, *Body Stories*, discusses the three languages of the body with which the therapist must become familiar; one of them is the 'dyadic body language'. This is a pre-Oedipal and pre-verbal language expressed in embodied physical phenomena in the treatment process.

DOI: 10.4324/9781003309048-12

Case description

Ron, a young man in his twenties, came to therapy at his mother's recommendation, the background being a crisis he experienced in his romantic relationship. His partner at that time had undergone ongoing sexual assault during her childhood, and relations with her were highly influenced by this trauma. Ron found himself on uncertain ground in a tumultuous relationship filled with destruction and violence, harm and betrayal, and felt erased and very hurt. Despite having separated from his partner, he was still immersed in much suffering and did not stop loving her and missing her. Ron's previous romantic partner had also undergone sexual abuse in her childhood and their relationship had attributes of violation, including threats of suicide, violence, and a constant presence of guilt and blame.

Ron is an only child of parents who split up when he was a toddler. The relationship with his biological father was severed for several years during his childhood because – according to Ron – his father's new spouse created distance between them; however, the relationship was revived during his adolescence. Ron's mother remarried a man who was a father to him and with whom he spent many hours and days. His mother was responsible for the family's income and was mostly out of the house, working. Around Ron's adolescence, his stepfather left. According to Ron, the separation from her husband was very difficult for his mother. He was angry that his stepfather chose to leave the family precisely at the time when his mother most needed emotional support and help with her livelihood. Because of this, he decided to sever the relationship with his stepfather. This separation from his stepfather occurred at the same time as a natural process of separation was taking place, but it turned into a rift, and to an intense and protective connection with his mother. Ron has positive memories of his relationship with his stepfather: shared recreation, sports, and trips. Along with these, there are harsh memories, such as unceasing pressure to become a 'man' and not to 'whine', so much so that it was an experience of emotional terror. He was pressured to detach from his feelings, and to push the limits of his physical and mental abilities. As this was happening, his mother did not protect him from his stepfather's Spartan ways and she was not present in the home. In the period following the separation from his stepfather, his mother had other partners, some in monogamous relationships and others as part of polyamorous relations.

Dance Movement Therapy (DMT) views the infant's primal relationship with the world in terms of an experiential and sensory experience. In parallel, the dance-movement therapist's body responds in countertransference which is, first and foremost, physical and kinaesthetic. The physical sensory dimension exists in every therapeutic process, but in DMT it is central and appears before the emotional experience is identified (Ben-Asher & Koren, 2002). In the treatment sessions with Ron, traumatic relationships were expressed through 'memory clusters' (Shahar-Levy, 2004) of disgust, sent as physical signals from the depth of his soul. Through the years, I have learnt from my patients that the experience of disgust is at times intertwined with the experience of sexual abuse. A body that is coveted, exploited, and violated in an irreconcilable sexual act arouses shame, anger, and rejection because it has betrayed, lost control, and disappointed. Additionally, the bodily fluids and secretions bond to difficult feelings and an experience of disgust. In their article, 'Internal sonar meeting of dance-movement: Therapist with injured memory cohesion', Ben-Asher and Koren (2002) present treatment that describes the connection between the experience of disgust in the room and the trauma of sexual abuse. According to the case description in their article, the dance-movement therapist's body absorbs the patient's 'memory cluster' which is associated with the disgust and it is transmitted to her in a sensory and physical manner.

The first session of Ron's treatment was filled entirely with disgust. Ron arrived looking dirty and his body gave off a bad smell of cigarettes and sweat. During the session he bit his nails non-stop, scratched at his skin and hair, picked off invisible particles from his wild beard, scratched wounds on his hands, and blew his nose non-stop. Following a number of similar sessions with Ron and in light of the ongoing experience of disgust and his poking about his body, along with my experience of a heavy feeling in the room, my sense grew regarding the presence of sexual abuse in his life, starting with the primal relationship with his mother. In answer to my question, Ron negated the possibility that he had undergone direct sexual abuse in his life and thus, the occurrence of intergenerational transmission of trauma conveyed without words became more of a possibility. As treatment progressed, the sense that he directly identified with sexual abuse that was not his own, and the experiences of trauma which surrounded him were transmitted by the body in the relationships he created. It was possible to sense the primal dyadic relationship which Ron experienced by the transmission of invasiveness and disgust during the course of the sessions.

When sexual abuse occurs, particularly at a young age, it takes place within a relationship which enables a distorted emotional connection with an adult who, instead of protecting and safeguarding the child, abuses him. For the boy or girl and later on, the man or woman, every experience of a relationship can be imprinted and stained with the content created during the trauma. In the case described here, the content is disgust and revulsion. I hypothesised that Ron's mother went through sexual abuse in her childhood, an assault which aroused in her disgust and revulsion, and produced the association between these bodily sensations and the experience of her relationship with her son.

The experience of a feeling of disgust arose many more times during the course of therapy: Ron would come to sessions only about half an hour after waking up, and at the start of the session he would regularly inform me that he did not manage to brush his teeth or to shower the previous evening after a long day of work. He would come to the sessions dressed in dirty and torn clothing, often mentioning stomach aches due to digestive difficulties and would regularly hiccup and burp.

During the treatment period, Ron's mother told him that she had indeed been the victim of ongoing sexual abuse in her childhood, and as a result, our discussion about sexual assault in general and the abuse his mother went through, in particular, became more open and free. Following this revelation, we could start to talk about the nature of the relationship between Ron and his mother in light of the trauma in her life, and about the way the nature of that relationship was affecting his identity as a man, about his choice of the romantic partners in his life, and the nature of his intimate relationships.

Ron is a young person full of good intentions: he is kind, polite, considerate, and it is very important to him to be 'good' and to increase the amount of good in the world. He splits off the content that is difficult, painful, and perforated within him and can express these things through the feeling of disgust. Ron lived his 'self' as repulsive and disgusting since he has never had an environment which nurtured him and was concerned about him in an appropriate way. Through his body odours, sweat stains, the dirty clothes with holes, worn shoes, smelly socks, wild and tangled hair, and the picking at his skin, an immediate and irritating sense of disgust and repulsion is created. Ron presents himself through these sensations and does so in a manner that makes him impossible to ignore, but at the same time causes rejection and thus replays the distortion in the relations from which he developed.

Many of the founding psychoanalytic theorists point to the connection between psychic processes, and physical sensations and physical symptoms: according to Freud (1923), the ego as 'first and foremost a body-ego', and 'is ultimately derived from bodily sensations' – 'mainly those derived from the body surface'. Reik (2014), following Ferenczi, views the appearance of physical symptoms in therapy as a return of early memories fixed in the body (Ferenczi, 1932). Winnicott (1954) fully credited the fact that the physical experience is the basis for understanding the psyche. Anzieu (1985) writes of the smell envelope as marking territory and as an expression of aggressiveness and sexuality in the therapy room. Bick (1968) attributes critical importance to skin which serves as a container for the body and as the surface for communication between the mother and infant in the first months of life. According to her, proper development of the psychic skin is essential for validating the boundaries of the body and the self, and for developing an internal sense of containment for psychic life. Abuse early in life which is related to traumatic separation, primal fears, and intolerable psychic pain is recorded in the psyche as internal images and feelings of perforated, torn, and injured skin, and transform the psychic skin (container) from one of well-being into one of suffering. McDougall (1989) speaks of the body-mind relationship and of the mother-child relationship which is manifest through the body. In her view, the self embodies hidden dramas created in childhood, which have significant influence on the adult person's life and body. Shahar-Levy (2004) articulates the concept of 'primal memory clusters', which expresses the collection of tactile and visual records of the world to which the infant's pre-verbal sensations are added. The connection psychoanalytic theory makes between psychic processes and psychical sensations is clearly expressed in the encounter with Ron.

As the therapeutic relationship with Ron deepened, I learned to recognise the days when he came to the session after meeting with his mother. In these sessions, his physical appearance in the room was powerful. I learned to listen to his body and came to know that his bodily sensations which communicate with the experience of general disorganisation and deep confusion attest to his being 'invaded', 'merged', and losing his boundaries, in contrast to other sessions to which he arrived more gathered and whole. As therapy progressed, I turned his attention to the relationship that exists between the content that was coming up in therapy and the body's actions in the room: every time we discussed his relations with his mother he immediately began to pick at his body, to open wounds in his skin, to scratch and blow his nose, bite his nails, etc. We spoke about the possibility that he was latching on to his body in order to feel that he exists and to signal his physical and psychic boundaries to himself, considering the sense of perforation in the envelope in which he lives.

I frequently found myself having difficulty in being in the room in light of the disgust which invaded me. During one of the sessions, while sitting and discussing his relationship with his mother, Ron tilted his body to the side and passed wind. After several seconds I managed to recover from the stasis that took hold of me, from the sense of surprise and embarrassment and I turned his attention to the event that had just occurred in the room. Ron immediately apologised and explained that he was not paying attention to what he had just done and that it was done inoffensively, with a lack of awareness on his part.

In her article, 'The Language of Absence and the Language of Tenderness', Gurevich (2015) explains Ferenczi's concept of 'identification with the aggressor': 'The other dictates to us an entire emotional value which lives within us and activates us from within' (p. 3). According to Ferenczi (2013), before the existence of the self, the infant's tender psyche is wide open towards the other. The infant has no introversion mechanisms and he therefore communicates with his environment on a broader surface area than the adult, and experiences it without regulation and filters. The infant has a tendency to imitation and immediate and automatic adaptation to the environment. In other words, the external is 'swallowed' up. An external assault at the tender stage arouses helplessness and forced identification and therefore, the parent has the responsibility to soften for the infant the experiences of the environment. In the relationship with Ron, the experience which presents in the room is one of blurring between the external and internal to the point of a complete non-distinction between them. He does not understand when processes within his body are seen and felt external to his body and does not understand their effect on the environment.

In a situation of 'identification with the aggressor' there is the effect of the external on the tender psyche which is not able to contain the aggression and defend itself against it, and so in order to survive, it immediately adjusts to the external by extinguishing the self (Gurevich, 2014). In a similar manner, Ron's identification with the aggressor is a forced identification through self-nullification: Ron is unable to set boundaries for his mother and his girlfriends, and the feeling he conveys is one of placation and self-erasure, along with the frustration and depression he experiences as a result. Ferenczi (1932) stresses the need for development within interpersonal relations and the importance of adapting the environment to the child's needs for tenderness. Balint (1968) adds that behaviours inappropriate to the developmental needs of the infant constitute traumatic factors which distort the personality.

It would appear that the adjustment to Ron's primal physical and psychic needs was challenging for his parents. The lack of boundaries and the 'confusion of the tongues' (Ferenczi, 1949) in Ron's life find expression in the non-adaptive relations between him and his mother who used him for her needs in the most extensive manner, and exposed him prematurely to adult sexuality. In their relationship, Ron is sometimes perceived as a child and at other times as a mature man. During the course of therapy, his mother separated from several different romantic partners. When such a break-up occurred, she would ask him to drop everything and come be with her. Because of the difficulty she experienced, she felt that she was in need of his comforting presence, and he would respond to her requests immediately, without delay. When his mother felt anxious, she asked him to sit with her and hold her hand until she fell asleep in his embrace and he would then transfer her to her bed, cover her and see to it that she slept soundly. During his childhood and adolescence, on cold winter nights, his mother would get into bed with him when she was afraid of lightning and thunder. In the not too distant past, his mother would come into his room in the mornings without his permission and wake him with a cup of coffee in bed. At other times, she would ask him to leave the house because his male presence was threatening to her women friends whom she was hosting at the time. In the past, she would meet with her boyfriends in the house and would ask Ron not to return home until her romantic liaison was over. In these situations,

Ron would wait at night for long hours outside his home until he was permitted to return, understanding that his mother was, during that time, engaging in sexual relations. His mother demanded that he be considerate of her need for space and that she could not be intimate with a partner when he was in the house, and this explanation was acceptable to him.

The shifts in relations, between being a good boy and being a threatening man, confused Ron greatly and in the main, neutralised any desire and ability he had for individuality. This pendulum, swinging between the experience of his self as a man and as a boy, continued for a long period until one evening, while sitting together in the lounge of their home, Ron found himself witness to intimate relations taking place between his mother and her friends, a man and a woman. This defining moment was experienced as a shock, wordlessly, and was later brought to therapy in a detached way. The look on my face when he told me about the experience apparently gave him the validation he needed in order to connect between his internal and external worlds. In the subsequent sessions, we could attach words to this destabilising experience and thus, the movement towards separation, independence, and leaving home had begun. Ron was very anxious about his mother's reaction to his 'abandonment' of her until he succeeded in finally leaving and renting an apartment for himself. As the therapy progressed, Ron learned to set effective external limits for his mother: he began to inform her ahead of time of his visits, along with advance warning that at the end of the evening he would not be transferring her to her bed. At the same time, his mother returned to a monogamous relationship and her new partner moved in with her.

Ferenczi (1932) coined the phrase 'the terrorism of suffering'. Berman (2014) writes about people for whom being a victim is the centre of their world, and for whom the victim identity becomes dominant in their relationships, especially with people close to them, such that the insatiable longing for compensation leads to frequent complaints regarding the lack of sufficient effort on the part of their close environment. Ron was raised to be empathic and to be meticulous about showing great sensitivity to his mother. As he felt it, if he wasn't attentive enough to her needs, there was the risk of incurring a big surge of rage or an anxiety attack. If he would 'hurt' her in any way, angry phone calls from close family members would immediately ensue, demanding that he be more considerate of her. Ron learned to nullify his self in favour of his mother's suffering, to placate her and to be considerate of her to the point of completely erasing his needs. His mother's rage ruled the home, and it was very difficult to stand up to her and set boundaries because she was 'ill'.

The mother's illness was discovered close to the time of her separation from Ron's stepfather. It is possible that her seizures which did not respond to medication were actually dissociative seizures which were misdiagnosed. A dynamic of guilt, blame, and rage dominated the home, as well as the repeated use of rationalisations whose conclusions always were that he must be considerate of his mother. Ron's biological parents taught him to use soft drugs when he was a teenager 'so that he would experience his first time with them', despite the fact that they were not of interest to him during that period. Today, he uses soft drugs on a daily basis and cannot seem to reduce the amounts. Ron's mother uses drugs regularly as a way to treat the seizures she experiences, and she has great anger towards the establishment which, according to her, does not recognise her illness and does not supply her with the drug. In the past, they would use the drugs together and it was Ron's job to supply them.

Through treating Ron, I can assume that the traumas in his mother's life caused her to experience significant parts of her psyche as dead. To hold on to life, she draws strength, emotion, and vitality from her son, while her void and stasis are transferred to him and turn into 'black holes' (Eshel, 1998). It is possible that these 'black holes' are also seen and felt in the room through the incessant picking at his skin and its perforation. Ron recreates and experiences the 'black holes' that opened up in his psyche and skin (Bick, 1968) through his unceasing preoccupation with his body. Psychic deadness (Eigen, 2004) is expressed by his lack of will and ability to advance in his life, to plan his future and to dislodge himself from his death-dealing daily routine. Ron is unable to find a job that satisfies him in terms of interest, ability to advance, and salary, this despite him performing his non-professional work industriously, persevering in it and working for many hours. When he returns home at the end of the work day, at a late hour, he generally falls asleep only towards morning and therefore does not have enough time to shower or to cook for himself, and he sleeps for only a few hours. Because of his difficulty in getting organised and studying, advanced studies are not on Ron's horizon and his future is unclear to him. In the past, attempts were made to help him in this regard but he fails to get the help and continues in an endless cycle of dissatisfaction and of simply surviving.

At one of our first sessions, Ron expressed great rage concerning his life. He described difficulty in working many hours at a job he disliked and had a feeling of social isolation, pain due to the break up with his partner and mainly, great frustration owing to the fact that his mother controlled his life and steered him as her needs dictated. His mother's invasiveness in their relations, her refusal to accept the boundaries he set, along with the demand that he be considerate, obedient, and devoted, brought him to the point of great rage which erupted from him in a shout. I suggested that he walk around the room and give place to the emerging feeling by using the punching bag hung in the room. Ron accepted my suggestion and hit the bag hard a number of times. The feeling was that a great surge of fury surfaced, absolutely overwhelming him and frightening him to the point where he had to immediately stop; the panic was clearly visible on his face.

At the next session, he related that he continued to feel the anger in the days following the session and found himself running in the fields, shouting, and throwing stones. We talked about the feeling of release he experienced alongside the great panic that arose, and from there about the perception of anger in his family. Ron has difficulty making the separation between feelings of anger and rage and physical violence. His mother is a prominent activist against violence in society and the atmosphere at home does not allow him to express anger and aggressiveness. The place of expressing frustration and rage is reserved exclusively for his mother, and his feeling is that he must be constantly vigilant so as not to become violent, particularly because he is a 'man' and perceived to already possess this tendency. In following sessions, Ron refused to use the punching bag and I did not insist upon it in view of his placating behaviour patterns. Phantasies of destruction and violence continued to be expressed in the room especially through shouting: 'I'd like to bang Mum on the head with a frying pan', 'to take an electric saw and cut off her head'. Ron would regularly examine my reaction to these declarations in order to check whether I was shocked by his rage. When he saw that the separation between emotion and action was clear to me and I do not react with panic to his words, he continued to describe what he would like to do to her. This movement of verbal phantasies expressed in shouts in the context of his mother continued for a long time but became more moderate throughout the therapy.

In one of the sessions, a moment before it ended, Ron brought up a ball of phlegm and rolled it around on his tongue. Before I had a chance to think and react, a wave of disgust overwhelmed me and I felt bile rising from my stomach. I apologised to him, rushed to leave the room and found myself vomiting. Ron understood that something had happened, looked stunned when I returned to the room and apologised to me. I felt something significant was happening in our relations and in contrast to the haziness familiar to him in his life, it was important to me to assign words to what had happened just now in reality. Before we parted, we managed to recap the session, validate what happened, and to look directly at one another. This was, in my understanding, a defining moment in therapy. After much time containing the disgust in the room, my body reached the limit with this and in effect, helped Ron set a boundary to disgusting content that was churning within him.

In the next session, to my surprise, Ron arrived with his hair cut, clean, kempt, and smiling and immediately told me that when he left the previous session, he asked his mother to cut his hair. When we discussed the event, he repeated that he was very sorry and that he understood that I was 'sensitive like his mother', and more than that he could not add. It is possible that Ron was reacting in an obliging manner and took care to arrive clean and neat to the next session so as to avoid a recurrence of the event and to prevent an experience of shame and guilt. At the same time, it is possible that he was moved by having affected me in such an immediate and profound way. Turning to his mother so that she could cut his hair left us in a transference cycle: the relationship between Ron and his mother is interlaced with disgust and therefore, it is possible that the invasion of disgust into my body and its clear presence in the room through both our bodies strengthened our connection, and for Ron, refined the feeling which is seen, felt and sensed in therapy. It is also possible that the request he made of his mother immediately following the session expressed the split between the good mother who contains and cares for her son and the bad mother who finds it difficult to contain the disgust.

The therapeutic relationship with Ron began as a result of his mother's recommendation and was paved with feelings of disgust transmitted from his mother's trauma and from the absence of boundaries in their relations. The neglected appearance, the malodorous body, and the behaviours which included picking at and perforating the body reflected the perforation of his emotional envelope and the internal sense of disgust in which he wallowed. During the course of therapy we were able to openly relate to these phenomena and to create awareness to bodily sensations and functions within the framework of the relationship. Along with validating his difficult feelings, which he received during the period of therapy, Ron succeeded in setting clearer boundaries vis-à-vis his mother, to shift in the direction of an independent life, and to create effective options for channelling feelings of anger and disgust. During the last year of therapy, the bodily manifestations of these feelings almost completely disappeared from the treatment room.[1]

Note

1 Thanks and gratitude to Idit Yam for her dedicated and wise supervision.

References

Anzieu, D. (1985). *The skin ego*. Tel Aviv: Tola'at Sfarim (Hebrew translation).
Balint, M. (1968). *The basic fault: Therapeutic aspects of regression*. London: Tavistock.
Ben-Asher, S., & Koren, B. (2002). Internal sonar meeting of dance-movement: Therapist with injured memory cohesion. *American Journal of Dance Therapy*, 24(1), 27–44.
Berman, A. (2014). Post-traumatic victims: On the aggression of sufferers. *Sichot*, 2, 146–153 (Hebrew).
Bick, E. (1968). The experience of the skin in early object relations. *The International Journal of Psychoanalysis*, 49, 484–486.
Eigen, M. (2004). *Psychic deadness*. New York, NY: Brunner Routledge.
Eshel, O. (1998). 'Black holes', deadness and existing analytically. *The International Journal of Psychoanalysis*, 79(Pt 6), 1115–1130.

Ferenczi, S. (1932). Confusione delle lingue tra adulti e bambini. Fondamenti di psicoanalisi, 3, 1908-1933.

Ferenczi, S. (1949). Confusion of the tongues between the adults and the child—The language of tenderness and of passion. *The International Journal of Psychoanalysis*, 30, 225–230.

Ferenczi, S. (2013). Billiards in regular 2n-gons and the self-dual induction. *Journal of the London Mathematical Society*, 87(3), 766–784.

Freud, S. (1923). The ego and the id. In J. Strachey, A. Freud, & C.L. Rothgeb (Trans.). *The standard edition of the complete psychological works of Sigmund Freud (1923–1925)* (Vol. XIX, pp. 1–66). Hogarth Press and the Institute of Psycho-Analysis. London.

Gampel, Y. (2010). *These parents who live through me*. Jerusalem: Keter Publishing (Hebrew translation).

Gurevich, H. (2014). The return of dissociation as absence within absence. *The American Journal of Psychoanalysis*, 74(4), 313–321.

Gurevich, H. (2015). The language of absence and the language of tenderness: Therapeutic transformation of early psychic trauma and dissociation as resolution of the 'identification with the aggressor'. *PEP*, 21(1), 45–65.

McDougall, J. (1989). *Theatres of the body: Psychoanalytic approach to psychosomatic illness*. London: Free Association Books.

Reik, M. (2014). The body of knowledge – The physicality of the therapist's body as ground for deep analytic work. *Sichot*, 2, 137–145 (Hebrew).

Shahar-Levy, Y. (2004). *From the revealed body to the hidden psychic story: The body movement-mind paradigm for dance movement therapy and analysis of emotional movement language*. Jerusalem: Shahar-Levy Publishing (Hebrew).

Winnicott, D. W. (1954). Mind and its relation to the psyche-soma. *British Journal of Medical Psychology*. https://doi.org/10.1111/j.2044-8341.1954.tb00864.x.

Yarom, N., (2010). *Body stories*. Tel Aviv: Modan (Hebrew).

Chapter 9

'Ground Zero Moments'

The Transformative Moments in Movement and in the Experience of the Mind

Yifat Shalem-Zafari

Introduction

This chapter proposes unique concepts for describing emotional processes in movement: 'simple movement', 'the ground zero moment', 'the dominant axis of the movement', and 'the step archetype'. This chapter introduces these concepts and illustrates how they are used in the work of the 'step-work model'. A case description of in-depth work with survivors of sexual assault using the theoretical thinking proposed in this chapter, and as such, is an invitation to freedom to think new thoughts about movement.

The word, together with the body and its movement are, for me, a complete human creation. In this chapter, I bring personal thoughts and examples from my clinical practice, weaving in my own poetry, written following the human encounter in therapy. These poems set new thinking into motion concerning the function of movement in therapy. Reading the chapter may set out a path for a personal, emotional, and experiential journey. This journey requires agreement to think about treating trauma in non-verbal and non-articulated terms, nor those which are consciousness-based and driven from the outset. Embarking on this new experiential journey bids dedications not only of cognition but also of emotion, the body and its movement in order to experience the process and not only think about it from the outside.

What is this life, where another's memories teem within us?

What covenants have been signed between us and the world as we preserve the memories of our forgetful gaze?

What is the word's quest, if not a feeling in search of a hospitable home where strangers congregate in sympathy?

The ground zero moment

When we come to discuss movement, it is customary to relate to its two parts, movement along with gravity and against gravity (Shahar-Levy, 2004). I would like to present a new thought which relates to movement

DOI: 10.4324/9781003309048-13

as having three modes: the active mode in which the muscle works against gravitational force and has the essence of will/future; the passive mode in which the body yields to gravitational force, has the essence of past/ memory; and, the third, which is between the two parts and which I call the 'ground zero moment'. That is, every movement occurs in three modes which produce a continuous pattern: active -> ground zero moment -> passive -> ground zero moment. This pattern repeats itself during the movement.

In this part of the movement there is a type of equilibrium between the force exerted on the body and the force exerted by the body. That is to say, when acceleration ends and the moment before acceleration in alignment with the force of gravity begins. The moment at which the force which the body exerted ends, but surrender to the force of gravity has not yet begun. This essence is defined and delimited by the boundaries of the actions prior to and following them. This moment materialises when the modes of action – active and passive – 'reset', and at that moment the speed of movement is zero. Under these conditions movement is not visible but continues to exist since it has no intention of ceasing. This new place of zero-existence space does not grant visibility to movement and thus it is possible to confuse it with the concept of *'immovement'*, coined by Shahar-Levy or with the 'freeze' which relates to the absence of movement. However, the zero moment is the space in which movement continues to exist and constitutes a connection to an experience of inner movement.

Active movement, counter to gravitational force, holds the essence of the future, while passive movement, giving in to gravity, contains the essence of the past, of what preceded it (even if only because passive movement cannot exist without the active, counter-gravitational movement preceding it). These movements define the zero moment which is a rounded moment without a before or after, beginning or end, and as such, it is expands the infinite.

According to Bion (in Anguayo & Malin, 2013), the truth as a crystallisation, develops from the infinite. It has shape and can engage in formative movement only if there is contact with lack of knowledge. The infinite nature of the zero moment enables an encounter with the truth as a space of consciousness. In this way a space forms for coping with trauma without verbal processing. In his study of memory and forgetting, the anthropologist Marc Augé (2004) relates to three 'images of forgetting' which structure the temporal dialectic between memory and forgetting ('return' – the first of the three 'figures of oblivion', 'suspension' or 'tension', and 'beginning' or 'rebeginning'). In the context of the zero moment concept, the second figure, tension (or suspension), can be mentioned, which relates to detachment of the present from the past and the future. In the same way, the zero moment is detached from the future action and the past action. Here too, suspended presence is a temporary situation and serves as a 'relational, historical space concerned with identity' (Augé, 1995).

A characteristic of the zero moment also contains an aspect of Freud's thinking concerning 'free-floating attention' (1912) as well as the state of reverie discussed by Bion (in Anguayo & Malin, 2013), both of which invite being into spaces that have no clear boundaries, and ambiguity is the basis of their essence. Freud invites the therapist to free-floating attention, while Bion invites her to a situation of reverie, in order to 'enter' spaces that are not defined as a separate entity, such as the zero moment. In order to reach the zero moment, movement should take place in a calm state, in floating consciousness and/or in a state of reverie. One should strive to focus on details of the infinite 'is' of movement and to try and peel them off until fully stripped of them. This will lead to a return to the 'dominant axis of the movement', to a detachment from the familiar and to an encounter with the new and the becoming. I will call the movement dialogue between the action countering gravitational force and yielding to gravitational force, the 'dominant axis of the movement'.

The dominant axis of the movement

On this axis, movement preserves a creational memory of the action of division between the heavens and the earth and produces a connecting axis that enables an existential space for uniting contradictions. This axis is influenced by movement parameters such as duration, speed, intensity, mode, direction, rhythm, and flow. These movement parameters are reactive, that is to say, influenced by culture, society, faith, relationships, and life events. Corresponding to the influences they carry, they will set in motion the shape of the axis in the space. At times, extreme events will become fixated on the axis's movement. The dominant axis of the movement serves as an axis of becoming for the self and functions as a spinal column for what I call the 'step archetype'.

The step archetype

The dominant axis of the movement provides the blueprint for the step as bearing collective memory of becoming upright in the process of human development. The erect posture engages in a dialog with gravity, producing the conflict sequence between active and passive. In this process the body carries the tension between up and down, between earth and heaven in all their representations. To expose the zero moment, the active and the passive must be stripped of influences until they are left bare, so that only their aims are preserved as defining the zero moment in movement. The actions prior and following must shed the cover of the 'influence-bearing movement parameters', submit to the dominant axis of the movement and expand a primal space free of influences.

The definition of the zero moment, which has no definition in and of itself but rather by familiar actions, the active carrying the future and the passive, mixed with the past, is similar to the definition of the liminal space in architecture. This space is the space between, which comes into being through the defined spaces before it and after it (Roberts, 2015). This is a space with no definition of its own but is specified as a passage from the origin to the objective where the passage from one space to another takes place. The other definition of the physical boundaries of the liminal space leaves the aesthetics of the space out of its designed context and grants it new memory-bearing meaning (which contain the present) and opens space for new thought.

The unique quality of 'in between' space is present, for example, in the 'Butoh' dance by acknowledging the existence of the step which is between the steps, which is called the 'dark step'. The dark step is the secret which exists between the revealed parts, which even nourishes their existence (Hoffman & Holborn, 1987). The zero moment contains various qualities of the 'in between' space, as described by the examples from the field of architecture, in the infinite and in the Butoh dance. The zero moment also contains qualities which become apparent in the 'negative space' technique, familiar from painting. In this technique, the object materialises from the focus on the existing spaces. The defined spaces reveal the liminal space just as the visible steps define the dark step. The zero moment emerges from the familiar motoric context in which another definition of the physicality of the movement exists and where focus shifts from actual movement to the space between active and passive. It opens up a space for an experience for which there was no space to be experienced, for thinking that could not be thought, and for the self to be realised. The undefined boundaries of the zero moment as well as the liminal space and the dark step and negative space all focus on the in between space, summon an exodus from automatic thinking and connection to the unthinkable, to mystery and memory.

The unthinkable experience and the zero moment

The zero moment is the part of movement in which movement has no visibility and speed, but enables the traumatic moment which 'froze' to change, to receive its own dynamic, to be alive and not deadly. Seemingly, it is a static moment upon which gravity has 'no effect', but actually, an expanding action does exist, a place for 'an unthinkable experience' and for transformation of trauma. Winnicott describes the acute deprivation of the infant as 'primitive agonies' and defines it as an 'unthinkable' experience. The infant's 'primitive agonies' are intolerable sufferings whose source is in the difference between the significant figure and the infant (Winnicott, 1963/1989). Traumatic events are events whose intensity of experience cannot be borne and those which are unthinkable and correspond to the primitive agony. The primal fear is unthinkable, although it can be described through images of 'falling forever' (Winnicott) and of dispersion in space as a result of lack of envelope-generating boundaries (Bick, 1968). Kalsched (1996) relates to the 'second line of defence' which merges with the unconscious in order not to allow the unthinkable to be experienced. This line of defence is familiar to us as primitive or dissociative defences. He stresses that these defences preserve life for those whose 'hearts have broken' from trauma. Levy (2017) describes the 'black hole' as a space for unthinkable thoughts and as a space to experience the self. The zero moment is not only a space for the unthinkable but also enables a bodily movement experience that will lead to change with respect to the traumatic moment which 'froze', that is, here, there is a becoming self, forming out of a sense of life.

Relating to the social space which enables the assault and which 'cages' the discourse is also called for. It is a social structure with respect to trauma as unthinkable. It is possible that the 'zero moments' constitute an opportunity for movement of society too. The zero moments in social structure, as space for coping with trauma, is a broad and complex topic which necessitates special attention and as such, is not at the centre of the discussion here.

It is important to clarify that every movement, even the simplest, such as waving 'hello' or scratching one's head, etc., is built of infinite zero moments. Zero moments are found on the movement continuum, though, unlike the active and passive parts, require special attunement in order to be alert to them and to what is developing within them. In these moments when the internal-active and the external-passive reach equilibrium, an unfamiliar moment takes place and as such, affords 'unthinkable' substance a place where thinking is possible. The zero moment, the undefined moment, can be given life by the active and passive activity. Therefore, comprehension in its respect is after the fact. One can be in it experientially in the present and it can be attained actively. To do so, a delicate and attentive attunement activity is needed. Being alert to it in real time facilitates after-the-fact comprehension. It exists in and of itself while our knowledge of it does not exist by reason of it but rather, by means of the actions which precede and follow it.

The active part of the movement bears the urge to move (Chodorow, 1991; Shahar-Levy, 2004) and the passion which propels the future (Symington & Symington, 2002). The passive part yields to gravity and bears memory (the memory of movement counter to gravity). Like the memory, the passive part changes and is not committed to a reverse process on the active movement's track. The zero moment is the movement moment in the present without passion and without memory. Symington, following Bion, describes this condition as enabling the existence of the vague, undefined therapeutic act which has the power to separate from the sensory and enable understanding to occur through symbolic identity in psychic reality

(Symington & Symington, 2002). This is similar to intuition, which does not occur via sensory perception but rather through an inner and creative act of thought. I tend to relate to intuition as a kind of inner guidance. Its voice can be heard in 'simple movement' that enables being simultaneously in the three types of activity – active, passive, and the zero moment. (More on 'simple movement' below.) The concurrent existence of the three enables a three-dimensional view of reality which contains the unthinkable. The zero moment cannot be created, but there is the knowledge that this moment existed as a result of an understanding which occurred. There is an indirect perception of the zero moment and it constitutes a new reality for revealing the hidden. If this is the case, the zero moment is the gateway to transformation from sensory-physical to mental-emotional. This is the moment closest to the moment of creation in its new sense, free of influences. This hidden moment, which is bounded by its location between preceding and following, contains the entire essence of movement: active, passive, and what cannot be included in these definitions.

The notion that the hidden, defined by the familiar, contains more than what is visible is also revealed to us in the commentaries on the Torah. They say the white space between the letters of the Torah hints at what is behind the letters and the reference is to things hidden in the letters of the Torah. The white background represents the 'light of the infinite' which is not embodied in the letters since it is beyond the letters. Shinboim (2014) relates to the white background areas (the white fire) as constituting esoteric parts of the Torah in which what is beyond words is shrouded and as facilitating new understandings and vision beyond the revealed. Thus, there is importance to the awareness of the high parts of the soul, from where mighty healing powers can emerge for damaged areas of the soul as well. The emergence of the zero moment to the light by that which is defined previous to it and following it transforms it into an unmediated space that facilitates contact with that which words cannot contain, space to become an honest self, and 'encounter' with the 'true self' as well (Winnicott, 1960/2009). The zero moment can be considered a round moment.

The power of the zero moment is found in the yielding to its timeless roundness that unites the personal and the objective and invites the unthinkable to be revealed. The zero moment is potential for transformation from a physical-motoric experience to a mental experience. The 'familiar powers' of active or passive movement do not operate there and at the same time, it exists on the movement continuum and with reference to it. The zero moment has no existence without the subject who perceives it and as such, it meets up with the individual's deepest personality, what Jung called the 'self' (Robertson, 1992). The abilities, which spread out within the zero moment bring balance and organisation to the unconscious, similar to Jung's primary idea of the 'self' as the central regulator and organiser of the unconscious mind (Kalsched, 1996).

The zero moment and trauma

The zero moment is essential for regulation and organisation of the mind and thus, serves that which requires repair in severe traumatic circumstances. The zero moment is like the line on the horizon, which represents what is beyond our ability to see, and one must be in accord with its ambiguity and uncertainty which spread from the familiar. Submitting to a zero existential space can be frightening and paralysing but may also be a situation that activates the imagination and thinking and constitutes a source for mental growth and vitality. In relating to trauma, Kalsched (1996) emphasises Jung's statement that a violation of the inner core of personality takes place in trauma and as such, it is unthinkable. The zero moment creates a place for the raw material of the inner core to become embodied. The inner core, like the 'true self', is the enduring part of the personality (Winnicott, 1960/2009) and serves as a place for the unthinkable parts, which Levy (2017) relates to as needing a 'place for self-becoming' and not necessarily for self-awareness.

To demonstrate the zero moment, I will relate to a state of movement which exposes an accentuated and unique zero moment – the jump. It is important to stress that zero moments constitute a part of every human movement and in practice, build it and are entwined with it all along its movement. The jump is an action which begins with an effort of the muscle to push the body counter to gravitational force and ends with the body's return downward due to the force exerted upon it. The suspension between heaven and earth, in which the velocity of movement is zero, is the moment the body is not active in a manner apparent to the eye and likewise, the force exerted on the body do not receive revealed expression. That is to say, there exists movement without visibility, movement which holds the essence of the jump experience and contains beyond what is visible in the revealed movement. Magritte's painting, 'Castle of the Pyrenees', incorporates within it a disturbing incongruity and sense of tension, emanating from the contradiction between our knowledge about the world, in this case – the natural law of gravity and the information directly conveyed by the painting – hovering stone. This moment creates a sense of mystery and contains information beyond the concretely visible.

The zero moment is peeled from the visible movement and creates a space for motorics of the revealed absence to lead to, perhaps paradoxically, motorics of abundance of the latent presence. Within it, there is place for the should-not-be experienced and the unthinkable in order to sustain the act of self-becoming. Levy (2017) states that 'when the imagination attempts to fill the enigmatic vacuum, the thing that is so hard to think (about) transforms into a kind of mental generator which produces psychic processes' (p. 19). In the zero moment there is potential for something to happen which has no other existence, and it is the expanded space for what is intolerable to be experienced and thought.

Simple movement

'Simple movement' is a movement which traces 'objective motorics'. The reference is to mobility disrobed of the costumes of influences acquired throughout the history of the individual and humanity. Costumes will appear in the figure of imitation, internalisation, reaction, fixation, social and cultural influence, and so on. The primal simple movement serves as the motoric raw material carved in response to motoric parameters. Movement parameters are influenced by the encounter with the significant figures we have consciously and unconsciously mimicked and they react to life events and situations, and are conducted in line with social and cultural codes. These influences garb the pattern of 'simple movement' and are maintained in the individual's manner of comportment.

Every movement is comprised of influence-bearing motoric parameters which 'clothe' the 'dominant axis' of the active and passive parts of movement. These parts of movement define the boundaries of the zero moment. Each movement bears the influences of the personal, interpersonal, and collective stories and thus, holds history borne by the body. The poet, Yehuda Amichai, was wont to describe how personal history is present in all its glory in all our present moments when he described how in all our actions the child, the youth, the soldier is present (Amichai, 2004). In her piece, 'Simple Movement', the choreographer, Yasmin Godar, creates choreography in the spirit of 'Stabat Mater' with the audience's participation. She makes use of the collective memory of bedtime ritual which holds primal memories – of mother-infant relations and even painful memories of trauma and death – an image of the Pietà. Repeating the action enables submission to the movement itself, the attentive movement will bring about the ability to remove additional details and contexts which are not part of the 'simple movement' of the bedtime ritual. Godar uses the medium of a performance as a tool that connects the audience to its self and thus enables the audience's self to become.

The 'step-work model'

The 'step-work model' aspires to 'simple movement', separate from the movement parameters which 'inform' the 'dominant axis of the movement', the active and passive movement axis. Simple movement is the utopian return to the dominant axis of the movement without external influences on the movement parameters which bestow it with various costumes. That is, in the attempt to return to that which should not be experienced and which is unthinkable there exists an action of unclothing of imprinted influences in order to expose the simple movement. This is how we will discover the dominant axis of the movement which exposes what I referred to earlier as the 'step archetype', bearing memory of the human walking upright and living. This process enables surrender to the zero moment that opens the potential for self-becoming.

The step template holds the 'step archetype' and contains the memory of the process humans underwent to stand upright. The transition to walking on two legs grants form to the unspoiled template of humanity. The step, occurring again and again, enables repeated observation and a peeling away of the parameters that were influenced *en route* to the simple movement of the step. The meaning of the simple movement is the return to the step archetype.

In traumatic situations in which the familiar existential mechanism shatters, an active mechanism is needed to create a sense of holding continuity. Infants can move non-stop in order to create this sense which is experienced as a holding skin (Symington, 1985). Adults get involved in repetitive physical activities in order to sense the continuity of being (Ogden, 2018). In this manner, the repeated step constitutes a kind of holding based on the principle of this sequence.

The step's automatic movement serves as a fixed pattern in which the disrobing of influenced movement parameters takes place. The step is a 'defined' constant and calm, sustaining the desire for simple movement and is the anchor that allows a yielding to the zero moment. The aim is to maintain the step out of a 'simple act' in a framework of ongoing stepping. The stepper sheds the crusts of influence so as to stand 'naked' faced with himself, exposed, surprising himself, and at the same time, a witness to himself. The process of repeated walking and observation of all the details of the step lead to an unclothing of familiar/imprinted patterns of thought in favour of an encounter with emotional worlds. The repeated observation of the step facilitates the unclothing of increasingly greater details: motoric elements, contexts, content, free associations, personal meanings, memories, and even unremembered memories. Ongoing observation can turn into a type of self-analysis that enables the self to form and to think its self in a new way (Levy, 2017).

Preserved in the motorics of the step are personal and collective influences which were shed in the 'step-work model'. This process allows movement to form in a kind of abstract template. Reference to these abstract movement templates is enabled by the recognition of zero moments, during which the self can experience and think in a new way. The fixed template of the step is built of familiar physical and motor components which produce a secured space for separation from realistic movement templates, and for submission to abstract movement templates. This process facilitates the forgetting of the present self and the encounter of the primal, pre-trauma self. The disrobing of the present-trauma self opens a window to another self to return and develop and perhaps even for a primal self to find a new step route on the path of his journey to repair. This is similar to the Butoh dancer who aspires to 'self-nullification' in order to reach something deeper, so as to disconnect consciousness from familiar templates and enable a fresh observation. The goal is to shake up the dancer's consciousness and to create a fresh experience that will burst through the boundaries of everyday perception (Noy, 2013).

In the 'step-work model' I developed in my work with trauma victims, ongoing steps were chosen as a 'movement template' which possesses a fixed, pleasant, and calming continuity. It will bypass the traumatic response mechanism of freeze, fight, or flight and will hold 'simple movement' which upholds the step archetype. The simple movement template enables the self to form in the zero moment. The step constitutes a meditative action for the purpose of emptying, builds a fixed framework for the undefined in the simple movement, and this allows submission to the zero moments with no fear of evaporation. The imagination attempts to fill the amorphous and the thing that is so difficult to think (about) takes place within it and produces psychic processes. Levy (2017) notes that things that are difficult to think require a place for self-becoming and not for self-awareness. It should be emphasised that the zero moment is not a place for self-awareness but for self-becoming.

Finally, one can relate to peeling the step away from the familiar template of the step action and its movement by what 'appears' as a result of the submission to the simple movement, as a movement which expresses truth of the kind that is not learned (Cohen, 2021) but which exists in the step archetype and focuses on the dominant axis of the movement. The step is peeled away from its acquired motions and returns to the simple movement, to the source, to its preparatory steps, which are connected to the intensity of the self. The step as 'objective motoric', with no memory or desire, expands a space in its entwined zero moments for that which is beyond actual, visible reality.

In the step towards the simple movement, the zero moment that is revealed is a place for formation of moments in the present which bear past memories which should not have been experienced and are unthinkable. It represents a framework for resuscitation of dormant psychic areas and enables form to be given to parts of a whole. The recurring step and the observation of movement, sensation, emotion, image, thought, and more enable the self to be experienced, to become and to think itself in a new way. The zero moment is 'free' of influence and it is a type of return to the creation moment itself, to the stuff of creation, prior to the influence of the past or the future. As such, it carries transformation potential. This moment enables connection to a primal, primordial being that expands space to act in a new way.

The return to the influence-free 'simple step' invites the imagination to fill the vacuum of the zero moment with the unthinkable, to transform it to a kind of mental generator that produces psychic processes. This process encounters the revelation of the otherness of the object (Levy, 2017), which constitutes a source for psychic growth and vitality.

The objective of the 'step template' in therapy with survivors is to release the need to create forms in space and at the same time, to intentionally focus on presence, attentiveness, and alert consciousness channelled towards essence. That is to say, walking while continually observing the step enables memories and repressed meanings to surface, to experience the unthinkable, and grants space to the self to become, to think (about) itself in a new way.

The 'step-work model' in a clinical vignette

FIRST VIGNETTE: AN ICE CLOCK

Memories bereft of images for thought

Are collected

Like crab footprints in the rushing and receding waves

Mid-August. I open the door, the sticky heat envelops me and does not let up. Avital in a flowered dress, strips a Popsicle of its wrapper. I'm confused for a moment, turn a wondering gaze ... Avital immediately understands. She says: 'It's okay, I'll put it aside'. I think to myself: What does that mean – she'll put it aside? It will melt. But I understand that something beyond my understanding is happening and I must enable it to exist.

Avital collects the syrupy juice from the edge of the Popsicle and packs it back into the wrapper, places it on the floor, next to which will be placed the sandals she has not yet removed. During the last year we have been using the 'step-work model', therefore, Avital stands alongside me, I cast a look at the Popsicle which is indeed placed near her sandals; she says: 'Don't worry, it'll be okay'. We begin. Now it is Avital who casts stolen glances at the Popsicle. As melt-time draws near, Avital's muscle tone increases and the interval between stolen glances decreases. The melting process represents an externally defined time whose beginning and end are connected, and towards which Avital's body reacts. When the muscle tone of Avital's body is exaggerated and a moment before the step stops, I remind her of my presence beside her. The step does not freeze, but the Popsicle melts. With the next stolen glance, Avital will say: 'That's it, now that it's dripping out of the hole, I can relax'. I repeat the sentence, with a slight variation: 'That's him, now he's ...',[1] Avital says: 'Where did that come from'? This is the moment in which there is knowledge of the terrible thing.

In addition to the external tension which allowed the internal tension to unravel, there was a separation on the patient's part from motoric parameters that were influenced by the traumatic event. The return to the simple movement on the dominant axis of the movement and the zero moment enabled being with an unthinkable experience that should not have been experienced. For me, as a therapist, the primal origin of being was the glance and afterwards, the possibility to release the body to the space of occurrence and to myself experience the zero moment. I refer to two different, though related, appearances of a zero moment, one in the transformation from the gaze to the body and its movement and the second, in willingness to experience a zero moment in surrendering to movement of self.

> After you met him who did with your body as his own
> You went out to gather translucent bees' wings
> Stray dogs gave bark to your heart.
> In the witch's hut you removed his sting
> In his dying
> Seeds of transparency
> Sprouted on a bed of hearts

SECOND VIGNETTE: TO AGAIN WALK TOWARDS

> Here lie our breaths on my contracted body and your hardening body
>
> Your exhalation encompasses my goose-fleshed nape
>
> The beating of our frightened hearts in the background, was it horror or an illicit moment?

During the Second World War, Jewish children were hidden in houses, farms, and institutions such as orphanages in order to save them from extermination. One, who in the Second World War, was a hidden child and succeeded in achieving a full life, marriage, family, and career – fell. Freedom of movement was stolen from her and symptoms arose such as vomiting with any sign of intimacy. This was the reason she came to therapy and immediately the question arose: did it happen or not?

> ... she walks, shedding one layer after another, the 'simple step' awaits exposure, like an archaeological find in an excavated mound. At times,

memories hidden within it are revealed. Momentary attention to the gentle curve of the chest alerts the arms to envelop it as if embracing an imaginary infant. Her breathing changes, a sense of life and confidence overwhelm her and she gives words to the moment, '... I am not alone ...' Her little sister, just born, is embraced within the arms of the 14 year-old. Safe, rounded and soft, she continues to walk. Her gaze is sent far to the tree seen from the window ... the time between each step lengthens, the muscles constrict, threaten to stop her movement. I join alongside for the walk, in a maternal gesture, ask her to together maintain the 'simple movement' ... the step does not stop ... the archaeology brush removes the soil from the six-year old girl squeezed into the double wall with her father as the dogs outside bark. From the tiny crack the splendid tree is revealed which, every morning, lost another branch to be recruited in the struggle against the snowy winter. What is that moment in which body is glued to body, breathing in synchrony, the muscle contracted, the body hardens, freezes, a moment in which the heartbeat accelerates despite the lack of obvious movement by the body. Was it fear or a forbidden moment? The step returns and finds its internal rhythm. I stand to the side observing the new step that appears, wondering at its simplicity.

Resuscitating the experience of the moments and acknowledging it as horrible, the easing into unthinkable thought brings about change to everyday life, the vomiting reflex settles down and intimacy is returned to her life. The zero moment enabled the self to become and to think itself in a new way.

The touch of the leaf to the ground awakened what was forgotten with its fall

Heaven's teardrop absorbs the present's being in a time that already was

Work with the simple movement and the zero moment can be useful in Dance Movement Therapy. The 'step-work model' is a private case for work with the 'simple movement' and the 'zero moment', which I developed especially for work with people coping with trauma. The two vignettes demonstrate how an invitation to be in the 'zero moment', when the therapist is a witness and the patient remembers, allows the unthinkable to form in a new format of movement experience.

Note

1 In Hebrew, with its grammatical gender system, the phrase 'That's it, now it...' can, depending on the context, also be understood as 'That's him, now he's...'

References

Amichai, Y. (Ed.). (2004). Like at funerals. *Poetry of Yehuda Amichai* (Vol. 4, p. 149). Tel Aviv: Schocken (Hebrew).

Anguayo, J., & Malin, B. (2013). *Wilfred Bion: Los Angeles seminars and supervision*. New York, NY: Routledge.

Augé, M. (1995). *Non-places: Introduction to an anthropology of supermodernity*. London: Verso Books.

Augé, M. (2004). *Oblivion*. Chicago, IL: University of Minnesota Press.

Bick, E. (1968). The experience of the skin in early object-relations. *International Journal of Psycho-Analysis, 49*, 484–486.

Chodorow, J. (1991). *Dance therapy and depth psychology: The moving imagination*. New York, NY: Brunner Routledge.

Cohen, R. (2021). On the possibility of authentic movement: A philosophical investigation. In H. Wengrower, & S. Chaiklin (Eds.), *Dance and creativity within dance movement therapy: International perspectives* (pp. 35–46). New York, NY: Brunner Routledge.

Hoffman, E., & Holborn, M. (1987). *Butoh: Dance of the dark soul*. New York, NY: Aperture.

Kalsched, D. (1996). *The inner world of trauma: Archetypal defenses of the personal spirit*. New York, NY: Brunner Routledge.

Levy, I. (2017). *The passion of the gaze: Studies in art and psychoanalysis*. Tel Aviv: Resling (Hebrew).

Noy, K. (2013). Thinking Zen – Dancing Butoh: Thinking Butoh – Dancing Zen. *Machol Achshav, 23*, 65–68 (Hebrew).

Ogden, T. H. (2018). *The primitive edge of experience*. New York, NY: Brunner Routledge.

Roberts, L. (2015). The rhythm of non-places: Marooning the embodied self in depthless space. *Humanities, 4*(4), 569–599. https://doi.org/10.3390/h40-40569

Robertson, R. (1992). *Beginner's guide to Jungian psychology*. Berwick: Nicolas-Hays, Inc.

Shahar-Levy, Y. (2004). *From the revealed body to the hidden psychic story: The body movement-mind paradigm for dance movement therapy and analysis of emotional movement language*. Jerusalem: Shahar-Levy Publishing (Hebrew).

Shinboim, T. (2014). The white fire in sources, art and therapy: On revelation beyond words. *Michlol: A Multidisciplinary Journal, 30*, 81–92 (Hebrew).

Symington, J. (1985). The survival function of primitive omnipotence. *International Journal of Psycho-Analysis, 66*, 481–487.

Symington, J., & Symington, N. (2002). *The clinical thinking of Wilfred Bion*. New York, NY: Brunner Routledge.

Winnicott, D. W. (1963/1989). Fear of breakdown. In C. Winnicott, R. Shepherd, & M. Davis (Eds.), *Psychoanalytic explorations* (pp. 87–95). Cambridge, MA: Harvard University Press (Original work published 1963).

Winnicott, D. W. (2009). Ego distortion in terms of true and false self (N. Naveh & O. Arel, Trans.). In E. Berman (Ed.), *True self, false self* (pp. 202–213). Tel Aviv: Am Oved (Original worked published 1960) (Hebrew).

Chapter 10

Whose Body is in the Room? One Question, Changing Answers

Orit Gross

Introduction

Childhood sexual trauma can, many years into the future, impact developing mother-daughter relations. Using a case study, the chapter describes moments of change and insight in the therapy process. It began with the experience described by the patient, as a life in which she has 'no body', and progressed towards the possibility of another existence in the patient's relations with herself and others.

The appointment was arranged in a brief, matter-of-fact telephone conversation. I knew nothing more.

With small, quick steps, Rachel entered the room. She wore a long skirt which restricted her steps, a black shirt with long sleeves, black socks and white sports shoes – she was covered from head to toe. Her face was pretty, free of makeup, her hair short, and only after mentioning that she was *Haredi*,[1] did I realise she was wearing a wig.[2] She sat down in a chair and I positioned myself in my chair, across from her. On her face, a smile fleetingly appeared and disappeared.

'I have a head, I have legs, and I don't have a body'.

This was how the first therapy session began.

A full body sat across from me. I tried to organise the head and legs of the 'no body' I was facing, I tried to understand.

'I can't bear being touched. That's why I came here'. In the same breath, Rachel continued and in detail, fluently describing three axes of distinct relations which brought her to therapy.

The first axis was her relations with herself. She explained that what was below her neck disgusted her. Rachel invested much effort in the attempt to ignore her body, not to see it and not to touch it. Talking about it was accompanied by facial expressions of disgust, revulsion, repugnance, and

DOI: 10.4324/9781003309048-14

recoil. Besides her head and her legs, she had no body and no need of it. At the next session she related that she showers with her clothes on, gets dressed in the dark, and her house has no mirrors – in order that she not encounter her body. As therapy continued, I understood the significance of the parts of her body whose existence she did acknowledge – head and legs. They allow her to disconnect from and ignore her body.

The second axis of relations is connected to Amram, her husband. Rachel, 28 years old, was married for 5 years already. She loves and appreciates her husband and the patience, caring, and concern he displays towards her. In her opinion, he saved her. Amram is the person closest to her and it is he who encouraged her to seek therapy. And despite this, Rachel cannot tolerate his touch. Despite the number of years they have been together, the thought of physical closeness and carrying on conjugal relations drives her mad. Though she is a Haredi woman, she does not frequent the *mikveh*,[3] the ritual bath, and in consequence, she thwarts, or in the worst case, rejects, the closeness between them.

At the centre of the third axis is Moriah – their eight-month old daughter. Rachel understands that her infant daughter needs her, that their closeness will grant Moriah a more normal and healthier upbringing, because that is simply the nature of things. But for Rachel, the matter is different. She would have preferred not to be a mother. On this axis as well, Rachel invests her energies in avoidance. Situations in which Moriah manages to get close to her and cuddle turn into intolerable moments, and end by Rachel distancing her.

Three focal points, three relationship axes with contradictory directions of movement and conflicting needs. Three souls, two of which seek her closeness, and the third, the owner of the body, lives in constant avoidance and distancing from the body she does not have. And all this is conveyed with fluency in a monotone and with dispassion. One sentence follows the other, with no spaces and with no breaths.

A short pause and immediately afterwards, Rachel asks whether it would be possible to treat the problem without delving into her past. I deliberated whether and how to respond and finally, I said that with her question she is perhaps telling me there is something in the past she prefers not to look at.

'Ok, so I'll tell', surprised me and she positioned herself anew in her chair as if she had at that moment entered the room. She stretched the body she 'does not have', opened her mouth, parted her lips and froze.

Tense silence dominated the room.

A long minute passed, Rachel relaxed and her body reorganized itself for the telling.

On the next attempt her body was also stretched out, her mouth opened, but not a word was heard. One attempt followed the other and all that remained was a tense body, an open mouth, and chilling silence. I had difficulty positioning myself in the chair, I debated whether to say something. I kept quiet. Stress, vigilance and anxiety took their places in my body. My mouth too, which opened in an attempt to understand what was taking place in front of me, what Rachel was saying, non-verbally, was quiet.

Long minutes passed and then it happened.

In the beginning, weak voices and chirps were heard, and then whispers, in broken syllables, fragmented words and lengthy pauses, in stutters and in a constricted manner, Rachel spoke. Broken speech replaced the fluent and focused speech I encountered at the beginning of the session.

After her older brothers left home, and in honour of her seventh birthday, Rachel got her own room. At the same time she moved to her new room, there began a pattern of repeated, inconceivable and unforgivable sexual abuse by her mother. Rachel began to stutter. No one was disturbed by this and life went on as usual. Rachel's life turned into a nightmare that continued for years. The connection with her mother and her family was severed immediately after she married and left home.

A pause for methodology: My intention here is not to depict the abusive mother's unforgivable and unthinkable acts. I am deliberately not elaborating on the intimate and graphic details, small or large, which occurred in that room – they are all horrific. The focus of the writing will continue to be the moments which took place in the therapy room.

The first session ended and with it my work for the day. Unlike other days, I did not hurry to leave the clinic. I remained in the room with sputtering and nightmarish thoughts. I remained open-mouthed voicing an unceasing, heart-wrenching and mute scream. I remained with harsh images of what had happened to Rachel, the little girl of 20 years ago, and with the difficult images of what is happening now, too, in the reality of her life in her home alongside her spouse and daughter. I remained with thoughts about mothers and daughters. I remained with thoughts about the abusive relationship she experienced in her past and the current damaged relationship between her and Moriah, characterised by rejection, distancing, and absence of touch. I remained with immense pain.

Rachel's question of whether it was possible to treat the problem without delving into her past also echoed in the room. The answer was clear – the past is here, present and shouting, and there is no choice but to find the way, through therapy, to look at it without coming apart. There was no option of fleeing from it or tossing it aside, it was here. The question concerning at me at the end of the session was whether it was possible to stop the intergenerational madness that was happening. I have no intelligent explanation for the speed with which I was 'enlisted' on behalf of the one who was helpless in this family – the infant.

'To open up here in the session – hurts. Not opening up – also hurts'.

Thus began the second session. Despite the pain, and with the pain, Rachel showed up and continued to do so regularly, always on time, for the next six months.

During the initial meetings, it became clear that Rachel's wish was to limit the relationship between her and Moriah and to diminish it in value. Time after time, she noted that Moriah was born for Amram, and so as to put up a good face. 'She was born so that they would leave me alone', she said. 'If she'd die it wouldn't be a tragedy'.

Rachel uttered harsh sentences, hurtful, and all were pronounced with equanimity. 'If she'd die it wouldn't be a disaster' was one of them. Even today, many years after it was said, it still gives me the chills. This sentence is incisive proof of the madness located in the space between the two.

During that session I did not ask Rachel who the 'she' was who could die. I was surprised at the intensity of this madness. It is likely that I was alarmed and did not want to ask. Every possible answer would be harsh, in my eyes. With time and increasingly getting to know her, I understood there were two options, valid to the same degree. If Rachel were to die, it would not be the end of the world for her daughter since the relationship between them was limited and very functional in nature; and if Moriah were to die, it would be a big relief for Rachel who struggled to not be a mother.

It would become clear that Rachel's great fear was funnelled into the moment Moriah would begin talking and call her 'Mother'.

'It's only a matter of time and it will happen', she said in great despair. And it was this moment she sought to delay, or to annul ahead of time. For Rachel, the word 'mother' is the epitome of catastrophe. In her own personal lexicon there is only one definition listed for this word – **monster**.

Concern for the baby's well-being settled within me and alongside it, concern for Rachel. Two lost souls. In my mind's eye I saw the 'movement' between the two – Moriah crawling and coming closer to Rachel's legs and Rachel moving away, ignoring her, leaving. The possibility of physical closeness between the two brought to the surface each time, the abusive relationship of the past. The touch aroused the monster that had lived securely for years in her body and soul.

During the seventh meeting, Rachel related that she insisted upon giving birth via a Caesarean section, completely anesthetised. 'To leave the body with them and go. They should do what they need to and I won't feel anything', she explained. The possibility that the infant should pass through her body and she would feel the process and be a partner to it, drove her crazy. She decided that the life which developed within her will not be a part of her. Only in this way could she give birth, only in this way was she able to continue to survive.

After the birth, Rachel informed Amram: 'Either I return home or the baby does'.

Terror overtook her. There was no option, concrete or symbolic, for the two of them to be in the same place together, no possibility of 'both she and me'.

Rachel returned home alone.

During the first weeks of her life Moriah stayed with a friend who knew a little of Rachel's distress and she took care of the infant. Amram visited her three times a day.

During one of the sessions I asked Rachel whether there was something she was ready and able to do with Moriah. 'To read books to her', she said without hesitating.

I was moved. A lifeline was dangled in front of me and I grabbed hold of it. I thought of an undamaged space wherein the relationship between them could exist, to become established and perhaps develop too. In my mind's eye, Rachel would read, Moriah would sit next to her, maybe get closer to her, and the stories, the pictures, the rhyming words would connect them.

I knew that a different kind of reading, a reading of a harsh text, a text with no rhymes or pictures would have to take place in the treatment room. Rachel would tell her story, the story not yet told, a story of horror and madness, a story that would be rewritten at every session, a story that needed to be forgotten in order to survive, a story which, just as it needed to be forgotten, must be acknowledged in order to live, and not only to survive.

Session followed session. Gradually, Rachel and Moriah's relationship received a place in the treatment room. The past had a presence without disturbing or destroying anything. It bided its time in the corner.

In the tenth session it broke through and took over.

In the space of ten minutes which seemed to me like an eternity, Rachel tried to speak. A storm was brewing in the body she had. She opened her mouth and no voice was heard. I waited and stood by quietly, hoped that the stutter I knew would be born, but it did not burst forth either. Her mouth opened and the body moved as if possessed by a *dybbuk*, a malicious spirit.

I told Rachel that I am here, that I see she is going through something, something which perhaps does not yet have words.

The storm did not cease. I told her that anything she says, anything that comes out of her mouth, no matter how harsh, does not mean she is a monster.

More minutes passed. Her body relaxed and then mine too. Tears washed over her face. Weeping was born in the room.

Crying is also a type of speech.

And after weeping, her speech returned. Rachel explained that the moment she thinks about her mother or is reminded of her, her body finds itself in an earthquake.

The memory which suddenly awakens and the thought which erupts from nowhere attack and transform reality, making it frightening and mad. The abusive mother within her takes control and takes on a monstrous and destructive presence.

When she was 16, following a particularly severe incident, she stopped eating with her family, kept to her room and ate only a few things that she snuck into her room. This went on for two months or more. Apparently, these were her desperate attempts to decide and control what entered her body, and when. Perhaps attempts to rouse her environment as well. The family doctor arrived for a brief visit, spoke to her about eating disorders and left. The world remained indifferent, nothing changed.

In the next session, Rachel related that she cried every time Moriah came closer to her or extended her arms to her, or touched her. When she read books to her, she cried.

In her weeping, I saw evidence that not everything within her had become petrified; in the tears that washed over her face, I saw a crack of hope, in her crying I saw proof that not all was lost. Just the opposite, something awoke within her, something undermined the inner distancing she had created, from her daughter and from herself as a mother. Her responses to Moriah's gestures and desires were not those she usually employed – imperviousness, rejection, and ignoring; instead, she cried. And that crying encouraged me.

And then, in an abrupt transition, with no dwelling or stammering, Rachel filled the room with abominable and disgusting descriptions of an all-pervading mother, about a monster who mercilessly bit into the body and soul of Rachel, the little girl. About a woman, controlling to the sick extreme, who cast her daughter's fate when she said to her, 'you are mine, only'. In light of these words, Rachel's statement about Moriah gains clarity: 'it would be better if she weren't mine'. (In Rachel's family there were five children, one of them her twin brother. As far as she knew and understood, only she was 'chosen' from among them all.)

That touch of the abusive mother implanted the monster into Rachel's body, a body she tried to escape from her entire life. With the birth of her daughter, and the fact of her being a mother, the monster within her was also born. This was the missing logic: as long as she does not have a body – she is not a monster. To acknowledge the existence of her body, to see and sense it, meant seeing and knowing the monster within her.

It is difficult to extract the monster from there, it is also difficult to leave it there – this is hard and that is difficult; and it is extremely painful. I told Rachel that I know for certain that in Moriah's eyes, she is not a monster. I emphasised that Moriah is not seeking to come close to her in order to control her or harm her.

Rachel listened to the words I said and did not react. And there was one moment in which I repeated to her that she is not a monster and she lifted her head, which was regularly lowered and folded into herself, and our eyes met. During one of the following sessions she explained to me that a look is also an invitation to penetration. This time she did not flee and did not rush to lower her eyes again.

Perhaps, with this look, a space 'clean' of monsters was born. Perhaps, there, a window opened from which she could see herself through my eyes and understand that she was not a monster.

Week 13 of therapy. Rachel enters the room smiling and before sitting down in her seat, said something was happening between her and Moriah. 'The distance is becoming smaller'.

I did not try to hide my excitement. Something thrilling was happening at home! There is movement, there is life on the relationship with Moriah axis. And as if this weren't enough, she added a sentence Amram had said: 'Finally, Moriah has you'.

I wanted to remain another moment in this new space, but Rachel decided otherwise.

With brusque rapidity, her smile vanished, and she lowered her gaze and disconnected. Rachel's body shifted restlessly in her chair, knocking against the backrest and then the armrests, as if it were trapped inside. Just a moment earlier, something comfortable and tender was present in the room and now, there was an extreme and shaky situation into which her body, and her soul as well, were thrown, and mine too. I asked Rachel if she prefers to move and sit on the carpet in the corner where there were pillows – an invitation to a different space, softer and more open, compared to the confining chair (until this session I had not proposed this option).

Rachel moved and sat on the carpet, leaning her back against the wall, the pillows beside her, and I with her.

Her mouth opened and she regurgitated story after story. Each story a thrashing, every event a whipping, things the mind cannot bear or comprehend. Physical and mental abuse, as the surrounding environment ignores them and keeps silent. Rachel's speech was fluent (with time, I understood that her stutter appeared when she told of events related to the beginning of her abuse. Fluent speech – when relating events that occurred at an older age). She spoke and her eyes closed. Her body spilled onto the pillows. Mid-sentence she went silent and did not move.

Terror took hold of me, a feeling that I had lost her.

I called her name and she did not answer. I moved closer. I would not touch her!

'What's happening, Rachel'? I asked.

This was obviously a senseless question, but nothing about this made sense: not the transition, not the disconnection, not the terror overwhelming me. Did I truly expect Rachel to answer me and explain what she was going through, as the ground beneath was shaking and she was beaten and bruised? The answer was clear. But my anxiety was also clear. I wanted to know that she was alive and breathing. I wanted her to answer me and reassure me.

And she answered.

Without opening her eyes, Rachel said she wanted to fall asleep.

I didn't want Rachel to fall asleep here in the room. If she were to fall asleep who could assure me that I would be able to wake her up? And, what had happened to her when, as a little girl and a teenager, she fell asleep, and in what kind of condition was she when she awoke?

Rachel's body slid onto the pillows (and there was no chair to contain and hold her). She fell asleep, fled her body and fled from me too. The past forced itself on the present. In the same breath, I said to myself that this was her way of showing me, here and now, how she responded to her mother. Two mechanisms – disconnection and petrification – enabled her to flee, she was not there during the abuse. To leave the body and flee. To leave the body in her husband's hands (who was by no means an abuser, but an attentive, sensitive and caring person) and to disappear by falling asleep or fainting or by actually escaping to the streets wandering about for long periods. But the explanations, as 'intelligent' or accurate as they were, did not calm me. And here, in the room, leaving her body in my hands and falling asleep? What was she leaving under my watch, only a body? And which body, whose is the body? And, in these moments, who am I in her eyes, an abusive figure, or a containing and good enough figure who allows her to sleep quietly without fear and who is responsible for her welfare?

Every now and then Rachel opened her eyes, and her pupils, as if they were frightened people, zigzagged from side to side. The eyes were like those I saw when I worked in a locked psychiatric unit. I hoped that Rachel could hear me when I said and repeated that she was here in the room, in a session with me, in a safe place. I attempted to return the present to the room, and to hold on to it.

I told her that she was in a 'safe place'. What kind of assurance was that? Safe, for what for whom?

And then she spoke: 'I'm afraid and I'm cold. Hug me, hold me'!

Hug her?! This was not simple, not a request to be taken for granted.

I understood that out of her intolerable chaos, in the earthquake, she was turning to me and asking me to help her. I was also afraid. I wasn't afraid to help, I was afraid to touch her.

The thought of holding her was as intolerable to me as the thought of leaving her there, a wounded animal, and not holding her.

'Hug me! Hold me!' She did not relent.

I told her that I was sitting close to her, right next to her, I told her that she was not alone, but these words failed in holding her. There were not enough of them.

To respond, to hug her? And what is the meaning of this touch? Who am I when I hug her?

'Here's my hand', I said.

I extended my hand to her and she clasped it. She held it with strength, she held me.

Silence within the room. I heard the ticking of the clock. It watched over me.

I was not able to embrace Rachel. I could not respond to her request to hug her. An embrace is a lot of body. The possibility of body-to-body contact was threatening to me. My body refused. My body safeguarded her, and me too.

Following this session, and during the remaining months of therapy, each time Rachel decided to tell of incidents that had occurred in her life, when she knew that an earthquake was about to bury her alive, she preceded the telling by asking me to give her my hand. Each time she asked – I gave it. There were times where I suggested to her that she hold my hand, and she took it.

At times I asked myself, where on my body did my hand begin and where did it end. I felt that sometimes, my hand began in my heart and other times in my shoulder, and occasionally in my neck and in my constricted throat, and every now and then, only at my wrist. When Rachel told of her first period and her mother's insulting and violent reaction, my hand began in my lower abdomen. When she told me of her difficulty with her developing breasts, my hand began there. And when Rachel told me of her running away from her house, about her disappearance for several days, about wandering the streets, my hand began on the sole of my foot.

My body was a hand.

And, what was conveyed to her and conveyed to me by her encircling hand, which was sometimes gentle and other times, tense and aggressive to the point of pain? And one time, my hand was so cramped in hers until I stopped feeling it. And at other times, the hand I held was that of a chick, helpless and fragile. And then, a complete turnaround, it was a hand full of strength which pulled me and drew me even closer to her. And when we get closer, where do we stop? Another moment and body touches body, and is the hand simply an excuse for another latent wish? In another second something else will happen here and I must protect myself, and her. Enough! I cannot go there. I am not her mother!

I was meticulous about ending the sessions on time. I did not change the therapeutic hour's 'rules of the game'. But at the end of the session, Rachel did not leave me. She stayed with me. She came with me into my home. She infiltrated my dreams, thoughts, she took hold of my hand, she chased me, and she was the monster within me.

To be held, to rely on, to look forward to a session, to want someone to listen to her and be witness, to understand that there is a connection between what is spoken in the treatment room and what takes place at home, especially with Moriah – all these new experiences, as good and important as they were, brought frustration and anger along with them.

I did not always understand her, I did not always absorb what she related or what she asked of me. And when I asked her a question, she thought it was because I did not believe her or doubted her words.

Sometimes I said things too soon and sometimes I said meaningless things. Sometimes I wandered off, in my gaze and thoughts. Sometimes I made illogical statements, such as: 'Maybe all the penetrations get mixed up all together'. And she was angry about the nonsense I said to her. And, if I helped her with the matter of Moriah, how was it possible that I wasn't helping her to get closer to Amram? And how could it be that I refused to prolong the duration of the session, because she's not getting anything done here! And she got angry, and it was all because of me, and I was to blame.

Rachel's anger frightened me less. The physical closeness frightened me more.

At week 25, I went on a planned vacation as a result of which, two sessions did not take place. At the session immediately preceding my vacation, she entered the room and I became worried straightaway. Her appearance told of neglect. She did not try to hide that during the past few days she had not gone to work (for years, Rachel worked in a nursing home for the aged). She said that she stayed in bed for most of the day, she said she had not showered, she said she ate little and did not read stories to Moriah. An attempt to relate what she was going through to my impending trip and to the cancelled sessions was rejected out of hand. Perhaps she was checking whether I would cancel my vacation if her condition worsened.

Rachel could not bear the separation forced upon her. This was the end-point for her. Decisive proof that she could not rely on me. Logic had no place now in our relationship.

I wished to leave for vacation with no superfluous drama. Inside, I was angry with her.

I left as planned and returned.

At the next session, Rachel informed me that she decided to end the therapy. Any attempt to relate to my vacation and what it aroused in her was immediately rejected.

'What has that got to do with it'? She hurled at me.

Acknowledging the connection created between us and its importance was impossible. Rachel claimed that the status of things at home had improved and this was the only reason for her decision to end the treatment. She agreed to come to an additional session. Maybe I hoped she would change her mind.

The evening before the session she telephoned and asked to come with Moriah. I agreed, after all Moriah had had a significant presence in the room. An hour later, she called again and said that Amram would also like to come to the session. This request surprised me. I left the decision to Rachel and said we would do what she felt was appropriate for her.

All three arrived to the final session. A couple and a little girl held in the embrace of her father's arms. At the end of the session, when they left the room, Moriah was embraced in Rachel's arms. I did not hurry to shut the door. I watched them walk away.

Six months passed. Rachel called and returned to therapy for a prolonged period.

Epilogue

There is therapy which, even after it ends, continues to breathe, grow, and develop. Almost two decades have passed since that first session. Many sheets of paper were kept in a folder bearing a sticker on which was written 'Rachel'. The papers helped me during the course of treatment. They were a protected and organised space that enabled me to enter and digest thoughts. I carried those papers with me to my supervision hours[4] which were essential and provided me with oxygen. Those hours enabled me to follow, step by step, the route the process delineated. It was a path that was long, painful, frustrating and at times, despairing, at times lost and disorientating, and for moments, enlivening and hopeful. It was a route with no shortcuts, a route that was travelled in the treatment room, the supervision room and in the chambers of my soul.

During the hours of writing about this case, Rachel 'emerged' from the papers. I saw her facing me as if it was only yesterday that we met in my clinic. I also encountered myself of 20 years ago (a complex matter in and of itself). In my mind's eye I saw the tree branches which came close to the window and knocked against it as I sat close to her on the carpet. I saw the bookshelf and I heard the ticking of the clock during lengthy blocks of silence. Physical reactions of fatigue and heaviness and nausea signalled to me during writing. And during the nights, Rachel found her way into my dreams.

Just before closing, I will sign off with a dream that appeared during the writing:

I am sitting with my partner on a cliff overlooking the sea (a place familiar to me, a place where I love to be). The sky is overcast and the water is dark blue. The waves are huge but do not break. In this part of the water, giant whales are swimming and at moments they look like submarines. The vision is hypnotic, riveting and frightening all at the same time. I decline a suggestion to descend to the shoreline and get closer to them, and I stay in my spot on the cliff, far away, observing their plunging movement into the deep, in and out.

In the dream I refused to get close to the whales (in Greek mythology, whales were the inspiration for monsters …). I kept my distance from them, a distance that allowed me to study the movement of their bodies and the movement of my soul within, like in therapy.

Notes

1 Haredi – Jews who belong to an ultra-Orthodox stream of Judaism characterized by, among other things, their strict adherence to the Jewish laws of modesty, clothing which covers many parts of the body to guard against forbidden desire.

2 Married Haredi women cover their own hair, often with a wig.

3 Mikveh – one of the Jewish laws. Following the days on which they menstruate, women immerse themselves in a body of water which meets Jewish legal criteria. Immersion is witnessed by another woman – the ritual bath attendant. During menstruation and until immersion intimate relations are prohibited and only following immersion are sexual relations between a wife and her husband permitted.

4 Gratitude and appreciation to Ms. Noemi Bronfman Huler for her supervision and counselling the entire way. Her presence was my anchor.

Index